Carol B. Pratt

Carol B. Pratt

Pacific University's Original Optometric Genius

David A. Goss & Scott E Pike

PACIFIC UNIVERSITY LIBRARIES
Forest Grove, Oregon

Carol B. Pratt: Pacific University's Original Optometric Genius

Published by Bee Tree Books, an imprint of Pacific University Libraries 2023

© David A. Goss & Scott E Pike, 2023
All rights reserved

ISBN 978-1-945398-14-8 (pbk)

Pacific University Libraries
2043 College Way
Forest Grove, Oregon 97116

lib.pacificu.edu

Published in the United States of America

Cover design by Grace Alexandria

Cover images courtesy of Jeffrey Pratt, Pacific University Archives, and Mayo Foundation for Medical Education and Research.

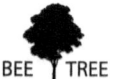

An imprint of the Pacific University Libraries

The "Bee Tree", an iconic ivy-covered tree that stood on the Pacific University campus for many years, was already old and hollow when pioneer Tabitha Brown arrived in Oregon in 1846. Mrs. Brown started a home for orphans that would grow into Pacific University. According to the Forest Grove *News-Times*, the tree was "said to have housed a swarm of bees who furnished the little old lady with honey which she sold to buy provisions for her orphan children."

Table of Contents

Preface and Acknowledgments   vii

Chapter 1   Carol B. Pratt, A Biographical Sketch   1

Chapter 2   Pratt's Examination Routine and Testing Procedures   15

Chapter 3   Pratt's Accommodation and Convergence Analysis System   35

Chapter 4   Pratt's Research on Refractive Errors   53

Chapter 5   Notes on Some Case Reports and Thesis Papers   65

Chapter 6   Stories, Tributes, and Perspectives   75

Appendix 1   *List of Tests in the OEP 21-point Examination*   91
Appendix 2   *Pratt's Examination Sequence*   95
Appendix 3   *Accommodation and Convergence Graphs Plotted by Pratt*   103
Appendix 4   *Pratt Accommodation and Convergence Norms*   107
Appendix 5   *Pratt's Method of Aniseikonia Measurement*   109
Appendix 6   *Carol B. Pratt Scholarship*   115
About the Authors   117

Preface and Acknowledgments

This book was written to preserve the memory of Carol B. Pratt, Ph.D., O.D., a highly significant figure in the history of the Pacific University College of Optometry and in the lives of hundreds of optometry students, and to create a record of the innovative optometric testing and analysis procedures he devised and the original research he conducted. It is hoped that the book will be of interest to persons who wish to celebrate Pratt's life and work, and those curious about aspects of the history of Pacific University or the history of optometry and optometric education. It is also possible that optometrists studying nearpoint visual function may find inspiration in the principles that Pratt delineated.

Chapter 1 presents a biographical sketch. That is followed by discussion of Pratt's clinical examination and analysis procedures and his research on visual function and refractive errors in chapters 2 through 5. Chapter 6 consists of some tributes and remembrances. Six appendices provide further information. Non-optometric readers may wish to skip the technical chapters and go directly from the biographical material in the first chapter to the celebratory entries in the sixth chapter.

We thank Isaac Gilman, Dean of Pacific University Libraries, for making almost twenty years of Pacific University O.D. thesis papers available to us and for facilitating the publication of this book; Eva Guggemos, Pacific University archivist, for providing helpful information; Fraser Horn, Dean of the Pacific University College of Optometry, for his encouragement and enthusiasm for this project; Lynne Olson, Director of

Operations of the Oregon Optometric Physicians Association, for information from their archives; Grace Alexandria for cover design; Pacific University optometry graduates Willard Bleything, Ted Dorn, Bob Edwards, Don James, John Rush, and Jim Weisenbach for answering our requests for their remembrances of Pratt; Stuart Mann, for providing four DVDs of Pratt lectures; Diane Goss, for assistance in processing photographs; and Larry Clausen and Scott Cooper for reviewing the entire manuscript. A special thank you goes to Carol Pratt's son, Jeffrey, for several email exchanges and conversations that helped to add details to the narrative.

Chapter 1

Carol B. Pratt, A Biographical Sketch

C. B. Pratt played a pivotal role in bringing an optometry school to Pacific University, taught hundreds of optometry students, developed new optometry testing and analysis methods, maintained a successful practice, and conducted interesting original clinical research. Yet, at times, it seems that his work is appreciated only by a diminishing number of former colleagues and students.

Carol Bert Pratt was the son of George B. Pratt and Carrie L. (Lapham) Pratt. George (1866-1939) and Carrie (1872-1949) were both natives of Michigan, and were married in Michigan in 1894.[1,2] Their first-born was George S., (1895-1977), born in Michigan; followed by Sadie (1902-1981), born in Arizona; Carol, (1908-1984), born in Portland, Oregon; and Norabel (1910-2003), born in Portland.[3]

George B. Pratt studied optometry in the early 1890s in Chicago.[4] He then practiced optometry in Arizona.[5] Some Native American baskets which he took in trade for eyeglasses while in Arizona are still in the family.[6] Sometime after 1903 he moved from Arizona to San Jose, California. But after the 1906 earthquake in the Bay Area, he moved to Portland, Oregon.[6] By 1908, he was practicing in Portland, where he remained until he died in 1939. George was a member of the Oregon Optometric Association and the American Optometric Association.[4] George was also a long-time officer and speaker for the Epworth League, a Methodist association for young adults.[7,8]

George furthered his optometric learning by taking a correspondence course from Philadelphia Optical College in the mid-1890s. One of the prominent optometry schools at the time, the Philadelphia Optical College frequently advertised in optometry periodicals, sometimes featuring some of their successful graduates.[9] This is what they had to say about George Pratt in an 1897 advertisement:

"Dr. Geo. B. Pratt, Phoenix, Arizona, was born in Michigan some thirty-one years ago. At the age of seventeen went into the book and stationery business, to which was added in a few years line of jewelry and optical goods. He soon found out by experience that no one should attempt to fit spectacles without understanding the eye and its defects, and therefore in 1892 he took a course in optics. After this he had good success in his work, but desiring to secure the very best there was to be had, he took our Correspondence Course about a year ago, graduating with the highest average, and later on meriting our degree of Doctor of Refraction.

"He writes: 'I want to say I am more than pleased with your Correspondence Course; every point is brought out in such a practical manner that I don't see how it is possible for anyone to take it without becoming thoroughly competent to fit the most difficult cases. Your Course was very much better than I had expected.'

"Dr. Pratt is a man of studious habits, and is achieving deserved success."[10]

Carol Pratt was born on December 23, 1908 in Portland, Oregon. He attended Jefferson High School in Portland and graduated in 1925 at the age of 16. He worked in his father's optometry practice during summers and sometimes after school, doing opticianry.[11] He attended Willamette University, in Salem, Oregon, where he completed his Bachelor's degree in 1929.

Just weeks before the stock market crash of 1929, Carol began work on his Ph.D. at the University of Minnesota, serving also as a Fellow in Biophysics at the Mayo Foundation. At Minnesota, Carol studied with

Charles Sheard.

Charles Sheard (1883-1963) held a Ph.D. in physics from Princeton and was on the physics faculty at The Ohio State University from 1907 to 1919. He was director of the optometry school at Ohio State from its founding in 1914 to 1919. Sheard maintained a close relationship with optometry throughout career stops at American Optical Company (1919-1924), University of Minnesota (1924-1949), Tulane University (1949-1952), and Los Angeles College of Optometry (1952-1953), and he published several important papers and books on optometric topics.[12,13,14] His list of 18 tests to be included in an optometric examination is seen as the precursor to the 21-point examination formalized by A. M. Skeffington and published by the Optometric Extension Program.[15,16,17] Carol's father George was a friend of Charles Sheard, and that may have been the reason Carol went to Minnesota for his Ph.D.[11]

Three letters that Pratt wrote to his parents in January, 1930 while he was in his first year in Minnesota still exist. The letters are upbeat and show a closeness to his parents, writing that he was enjoying his studies and that he didn't mind the heavy snow and cold temperatures that they were having. He wrote that he had attended a church service at the Wesley Foundation, but that he preferred the Presbyterian minister. He mentioned taking courses in calculus, physical chemistry, experimental optics, spectrum analysis, and radioactivity, and starting lab work with radium and x-rays. Optometry came up in one of the letters when he reported to his father that he and Charles Sheard had discussed the pioneering work being done in vision training by T. J. Arneson and R. M. Peckham.

While in Minnesota, Carol B. Pratt met Carol J. Adams, a Minnesota native. Carol Adams was a hematology laboratory assistant at the Mayo Clinic. She had musical talent and played the piano. They were married on July 6, 1931. To avoid confusion, Carol Adams Pratt and Carol Bert Pratt would become known to friends as Carol A. and Carol

B.[11] They had five children: Nancy Jean (1932-2004); George Byron (1934-1947); Susan Carolyn, born 1935; Stuart Carlton (1937-2002); and Jeffrey Charles, born 1949.

Carol B. received his Ph.D. in biophysics from the University of Minnesota in 1933. He stayed in Minnesota doing research and serving as an instructor in biophysics at the Mayo Foundation through the summer of 1935.[18] During that time, he published several biophysics papers with Charles Sheard.[19,20,21,22,23,24,25]

In the fall of 1935, Pratt returned to Portland with his family and began teaching at the North Pacific College of Optometry (NPCO) in Portland. He also took the courses for his optometry degree. In a January, 1936 letter to Charles Sheard, Pratt said, "I am again attending school, both as a student and instructor, and this being the time of semester examinations, I am in a whirl of studying, reviewing, preparing examinations, correcting papers, and so forth."[26]

In the mid to late 1930s, optometry school curricula were three years in length. At that time, only about one-fifth of optometry students had attended college before optometry school.[27] With Pratt's intelligence, previous education, and experience in his father's practice, he was able to complete the optometry degree in one year.

Pratt went into practice with his father in Portland upon graduation from NPCO in 1936. It is unclear whether Pratt continued on the NPCO faculty after 1936. He worked with his father until George's death in 1939 and then continued the practice in Portland until the mid-1970s. In the late 1930s and early 1940s, the practice was in the Alderway Building on SW Alder Street. In the 1950s, Pratt's practice was located in the Morgan Building in downtown Portland, a building which is now in the National Register of Historic Places. Pratt became a member of the Oregon Optometric Association and American Optometric Association early in his years of practice, and he was a member of the Oregon State Board of Examiners in Optometry from 1938 to 1941.[28,29]

Optometry school enrollments decreased markedly during World

War II, and as a consequence, NPCO suspended operations in 1943. NPCO had been formed in the mid 1920s through the merger of the DeKeyser Institute of Optometry and the Oregon College of Ocular Sciences.[27] In 1941, NPCO was purchased from its owner, Harry Lee Fording, by two of its 1939 graduates, Newton Wesley and Roy Clunes. Upon the suspension of operation, power of attorney for NPCO was transferred to one of its 1941 graduates, Clarence Carkner.[30,31,32,33]

In 1944, Carkner proposed to the Oregon Optometric Association (OOA) that it purchase the charter and possessions of NPCO, and arrange for their transfer to an optometry school to be started at a university in the vicinity of Portland. The OOA assigned Pratt with the task of studying area universities for a potential home for an optometry school. The OOA accepted Pratt's recommendation of Pacific University.[34] Clarence Carkner headed an OOA committee to raise funding for the purchase of the NPCO charter and the start of the school at Pacific University.[30] The Pacific University Board of Trustees voted to accept the NPCO charter in May of 1945, and classes started that fall.

Pratt became the first optometry professor at Pacific University in 1945, and for the first two or three years, he carried the responsibilities of Dean.[30,34] Faculty from other university departments assisted in the instruction of the basic sciences. Optometrists Clarence Carkner and Hugh Webb were part-time instructors at the start of the school.[30] The initial optometry curriculum at Pacific was put together by Pratt working with the science faculty and a five-member advisory board of optometrists. The early curriculum of five years total of pre-optometry study and optometry school reflected Pratt's belief in a liberal arts education, combined with a strong grounding in the sciences, along with the technical aspects of clinical practice.[34]

Pratt served on the Pacific University faculty from 1945 to 1974. He continued his practice in Portland while on the faculty. He was also active in the OOA. The OOA passed a resolution in 1953 thanking him for "his valuable contributions to the profession of Optometry," and he served as

OOA president in 1954-55. Pratt's wife, Carol A., was an active member of the OOA women's auxiliary from 1937 into the 1950s.[35,36]

Concern for the environment led the Pratts to purchase 80 wooded acres near Carver, an unincorporated community in Clackamas County, east of Portland, in 1941. Their property was largely undeveloped. Their house had been built in 1924. In the 1950s, they purchased an additional 40 adjacent acres. There is a labyrinth of caves, which the Pratt children frequently explored, on the acreage. A large portion of the property eventually became a conservation easement greenspace.

Pratt had the first of several heart attacks in March of 1959 after playing volleyball at the old Pacific University gym.[37] He returned to his office, but felt bad and had to lie down. He was taken to the hospital for a long recovery. Another heart attack occurred a few years later when he was walking in his woods with his son Jeff. After Jeff ran back to the house and called the Carver store where his mother had gone grocery shopping, the local volunteer fire department arrived to rush him to the hospital. A third major heart attack occurred in the mid-1960s at an Oregon Optometric Association meeting, again requiring several days in the hospital.[36]

Pratt's wife, Carol A., died in July, 1973, after a long illness of several years. During that time, her primary caregivers were C. B. and Jeff.[11]

It is surprising that Pratt could manage a faculty position, an optometry practice, family life, a long commute, and still have time for all his work on patient data and graphs. His son Jeff thinks that part of the explanation is that C. B. didn't seem to require a lot of sleep. Though C. B. was an early riser, Jeff can remember him sitting in his living room chair late at night poring over data, making notes, and plotting graphs.[36]

Carol B. Pratt died March 12, 1984. He made many contributions to optometry in his lifetime, in addition to those mentioned in this chapter. He developed a unique, detailed optometric examination routine (see Chapter 2 and Appendix 2). He devised a unique and effective method of analyzing accommodation and convergence test findings (Chapter 3).

He conducted research on myopia and astigmatism (Chapter 4). He was the advisor for many student research projects (Chapter 5). He came up with a unique method for measuring aniseikonia (Chapter 4 and Appendix 5). Unfortunately, Pratt published only one paper in an optometry journal.[38] His son Jeff thinks that his reticence to publish his findings may have stemmed from ill feelings as a consequence of a misunderstanding that he and Charles Sheard had with a Mayo Clinic physician over a publication on work done there. That reluctance to publish and his humility may explain why his name is not recognized by many today, despite the esteem in which he was held by colleagues and students (see Chapter 6). The following chapters may show why one colleague referred to him as "Mr. Optometry."[34]

References

1. Find-a-Grave index. www.findagrave.com.
2. Michigan marriage records. www.ancestry.com.
3. United States federal census, 1900, 1910, and 1920. www.ancestry.com.
4. George Pratt obituary. Optical J Rev Optom 1939;76(20):49.
5. www.christopherson.net/genealogy/familytree/lapham/lapham.carrie_003_1872.html.
6. Pratt J. Email to Scott Pike, October, 2020.
7. Conventions hold interest of churches this week. The Sunday Oregonian, May 19, 1918, p. 10.
8. Optom Weekly, Sept. 4, 1924.
9. Goss DA. Christian Henry Brown (1857-1933) and the Philadelphia Optical College. Hindsight: J Optom Hist 2010;41:114-121.
10. Advertisement for Philadelphia Optical College. The Keystone, February, 1897.
11. Pratt J. Telephone call with Scott Pike, October 12, 2020.
12. Newcomb RD. Our History in Focus: The First 100 Years of The Ohio State University College of Optometry. Columbus, OH: The Ohio State University, 2014:11-14, 165-166.
13. Koch CC. Minnesota honors Charles Sheard. Am J Optom Arch Am Acad Optom 1963;40:102-105.
14. Goss DA. Charles Sheard (1883-1963). Hindsight: J Optom Hist 2016;47:35-37.
15. Sheard C. Dynamic Ocular Tests. Columbus, OH: Lawrence Press, 1917. Reprinted in: Sheard C. The Sheard Volume: Selected Writings in Visual and Ophthalmic

Optics. Philadelphia: Chilton, 1957:43.
16. Borish IM. 21 points. Newsletter Optom Hist Soc 1987;18:23-24.
17. Hendrickson H. 21 points and more. Newsletter Optom Hist Soc 1987;18:55-56.
18. Mayo Clinic. Physicians of the Mayo Clinic and the Mayo Foundation. Minneapolis: University of Minnesota Press, 1937:1139-1140.
19. Sheard C, Pratt CB. Changes in temperatures of tissues after systemic applications of short wave electric fields. Proc Soc Exper Biol Med 1935;32:763-766.
20. Pratt CB, Sheard C. Thermal changes produced in tissues by local applications of radiothermy. Proc Soc Exper Biol Med 1935;32:766-771.
21. Sheard C, Pratt CB. The effects of short wave electric fields on the cataphoretic velocities of Streptococci. Proc Soc Exper Biol Med 1935;32: 899-902.
22. Pratt CB, Sheard C. The electrophoretic characteristics of Streptococci exposed to high frequency fields. Proc Soc Exper Biol Med 1935;32:903-906.
23. Allen RB, Pratt CB, Sheard C. High frequency electric fields and Roentgen rays: Effects on compensatory hypertrophy of the kidney. Arch Path 1935;19:502-504.
24. Pratt CB, Sheard C. The electrophoretic characteristics of Streptococci. Part I. Protoplasma 1935;23:14-23.
25. Pratt CB, Sheard C, Rosenow EC. The electrophoretic characteristics of Streptococci. Part II. Protoplasma 1935;23:24-33.
26. Pratt CB. Letter to Charles Sheard, January 13, 1936.
27. Goss DA. From Spectacle Making Trade to Scholarly Profession: A History of Optometry in the United States. Forest Grove, OR: Pacific University Press, 2022:276-277.
28. Blue Book of Optometrists, 15th ed. Chicago: Professional Press, 1940.
29. Members State Board of Examiners in Optometry and Oregon Board of Optometry. www.oregon.gov/obo/Documents/board/BrdMmbrs_since_1905_3_27_18.pdf.
30. Baker WJ, ed. The Twenty-fifth Anniversary of the College of Optometry at Pacific University. Oregon Optometrist 1970;37:4-25.
31. Wesley NK. Contacts – One Hundred Years Plus. New York: Vantage Press, 1988:23-27.
32. Fletcher SK. The College of Optometry at Pacific University celebrates its 50th year. J Am Optom Assoc 1995;66:599-601.
33. Miranda G, Read R. Splendid Audacity: the Story of Pacific University. Seattle, WA: Documentary Book Publishers, 2000:87-91.
34. Haynes HM. In Memory of a Friend. Handwritten copy of a eulogy for Carol B. Pratt read at memorial services at Oregon City, Oregon, March 16, 1984.
35. Oregon Optometric Physicians Association archives.
36. Pratt J. Conversation with Scott Pike, October, 2021.
37. Pratt J. Email to Scott Pike, February, 2021.
38. Pratt CB. The variation in phorias with time after dissociation and magnitude of

convergence. Am J Optom Arch Am Acad Optom 1962;39:257-263.

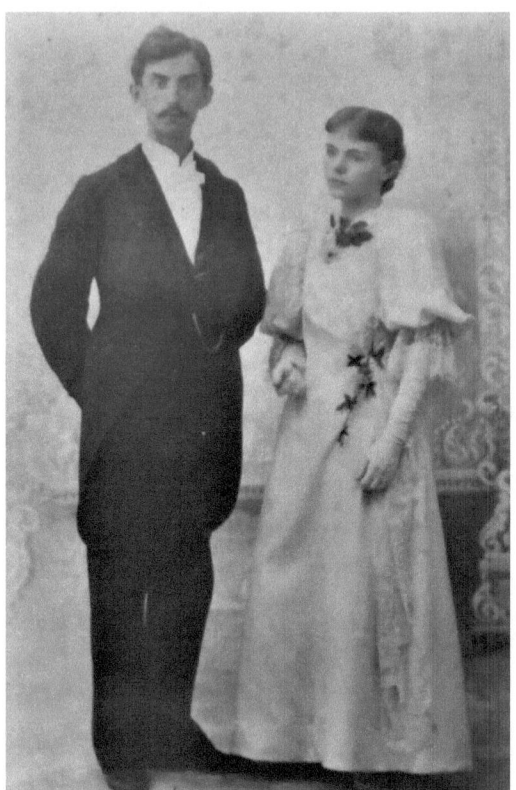

Figure 1.1. Carol Pratt's parents, George Pratt and Carrie Lapham, on their wedding day in 1894. (Image courtesy Jeffrey Pratt)

Figure 1.2. Carol B. Pratt's father, George Pratt (1866-1939). (Photo from newspaper article, "Conventions hold interest of churches this week," The Sunday Oregonian, May 19, 1918, page 10)

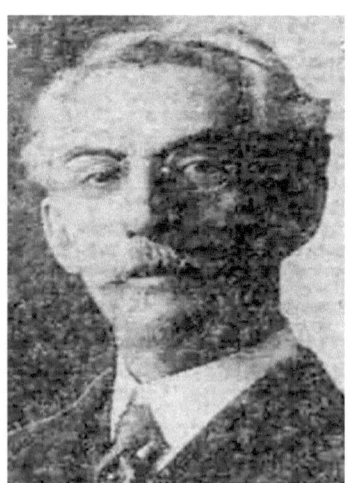

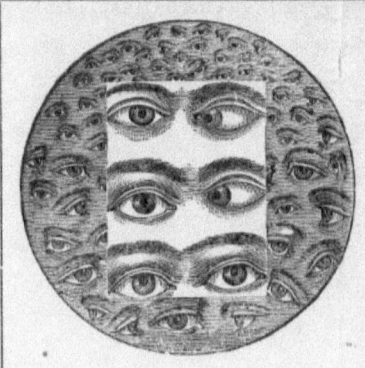

Figure 1.3. First page of a four page 1903 flyer announcing the availability of George Pratt's services. The remainder of the flyer consists primarily of testimonials from satisfied patients. He was referred to as an optician because the term optometrist was not yet in wide usage. (Image courtesy of Jeffrey Pratt)

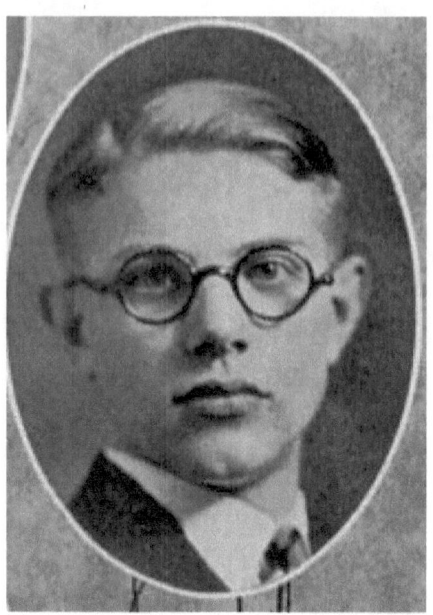

Figure 1.4. Sixteen year old Carol B. Pratt. (From The Spectrum, Jefferson High School yearbook Portland, Oregon, June, 1925)

Figure 1.5. Carol B. Pratt and Carol Adams on their wedding day in 1931. (Image courtesy Jeffrey Pratt)

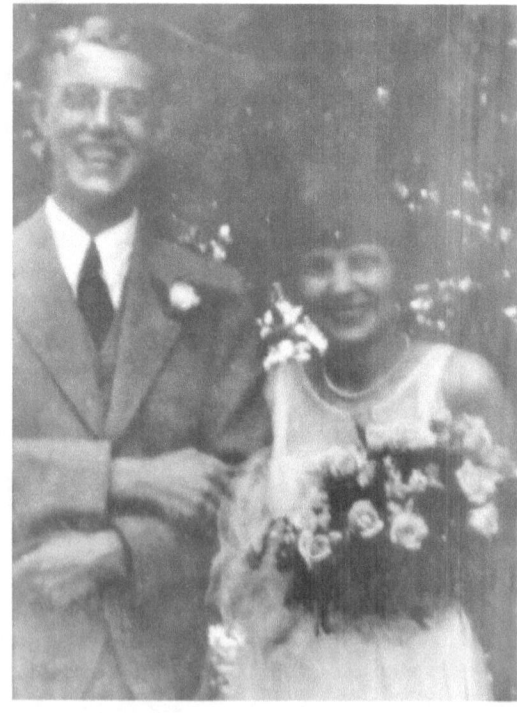

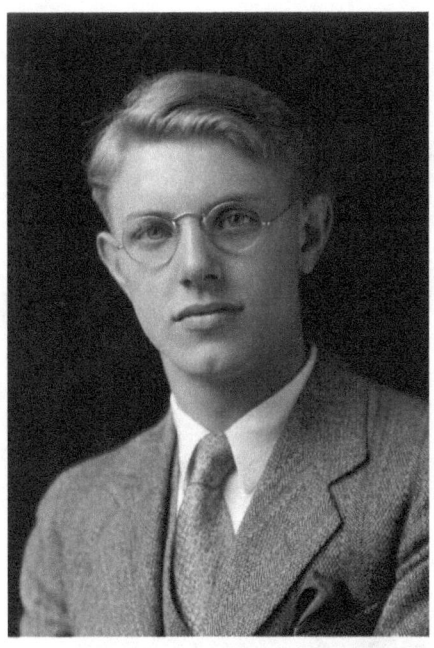

Figure 1.6. Carol B. Pratt in the 1930s. (Used with permission of Mayo Foundation for Medical Education and Research. All rights reserved.)

Figure 1.7. Carol B. Pratt, in about 1970. (From Pacific University yearbook, 1970)

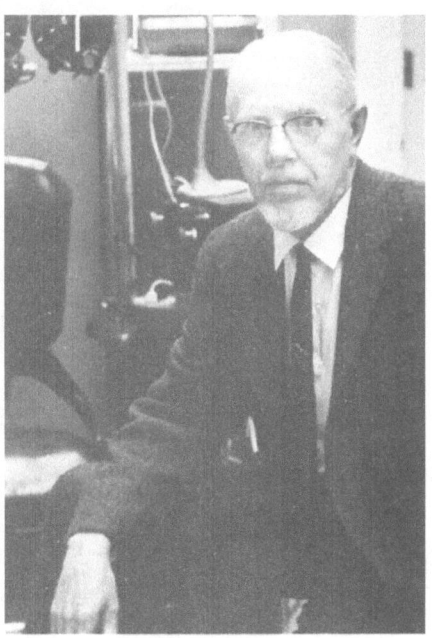

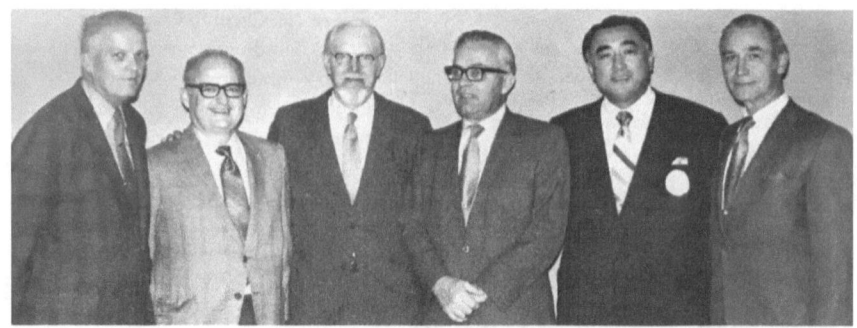

Figure 1.8. Pacific University College of Optometry pioneers, at 25th anniversary celebration in 1970; from left to right: charter class graduates Clarence Bondelid and Terry Pace, Carol B. Pratt, Clarence Carkner, Newton Wesley, and Roy Clunes. From The Oregon Optometrist, November-December, 1970;37(6):25. (Image courtesy of Oregon Optometric Physicians Association)

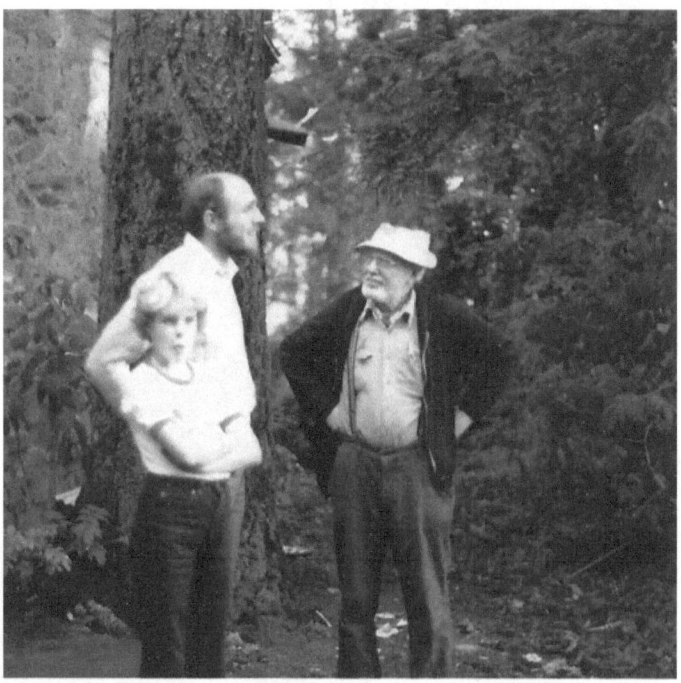

Figure 1.9. Scott Pike and his daughter Jenna (left) with Carol B. Pratt on Pratt's acreage, October, 1983. (Photo from Scott Pike)

Chapter 2

Pratt's Examination Routine and Testing Procedures

For about the first six months after Carol Pratt entered practice with his father in 1936, he used an examination routine that was essentially the same as the 21-point examination published by the Optometric Extension Program (OEP). The OEP 21-point examination came from an attempt in the 1920s and 1930s to bring order and thoroughness into the optometric examination. That attempt was successful, as the 21-point exam was widely adopted throughout the United States and taught in optometry schools for several decades. (see Appendix 1 for a list of the OEP tests).[1]

The OEP 21-point exam included static retinoscopy. Pratt found that he was not as good a retinoscopist as his father, so he sought to design an examination routine that would be "first-rate" without retinoscopy.[2] On January 1 of each year from 1937 to 1941, he made various changes in his examination and statistically evaluated the results.

He arrived at an examination routine in which near tests were done before far tests, unlike the usual testing sequence then and today. Although it is not possible to accurately predict the complexities of near-point visual function from the results of far tests, Pratt found that by the end of his particular set of near tests, he could predict the result of the far tests, including the subjective refraction. He was thus able to complete the distance refraction in minimal time. Pratt felt that an additional advantage of starting the examination with near tests was that accommodation and convergence function could be tested at an early stage of the examination when the patient was less likely to be fatigued or less attentive.

NEAR TESTS IN PRATT'S ROUTINE EXAMINATION

Pratt continued to make small refinements in testing methods and targets, but after about 1941, his near testing procedure included the following (Although Pratt did not then use the OEP test sequence, he generally referred to tests by their OEP numbers, and they can serve as a useful abbreviation):

- Monocular plus-to-blur-out at 16 inches (40 cm), sometimes referred to as the 21m or 21 monocular test because binocular plus-to-blur-out is test number 21 in the OEP testing sequence,
- Pratt near cylinder test for astigmatism,
- Binocular plus-to-blur-out at 16 inches (OEP number 21 or negative relative accommodation, NRA) and recovery,
- Unfused or monocular cross cylinder at 16 inches and phoria through the endpoint of that test (OEP test numbers 14A and 15A),
- Binocular plus-to-blur-out at 16 inches measured through 16Δ base-in,
- Fused or binocular cross cylinder (BCC) at 16 inches measured through base-in prism (usually 16Δ BI), with no prism (OEP test number 14B), and with base-out prism (usually 8 or 10Δ BO), each with a pre-set lens on the plus side and then decreasing plus to the endpoint (high neutral),
- Fused or binocular cross cylinder (BCC) at 16 inches, starting with a pre-set lens on the minus side and then increasing plus to the endpoint (low neutral),
- von Graefe dissociated phorias at 16 inches with various plus and minus spherical lens additions,
- Binocular minus-to-blur-out at 16 inches (OEP test number 20 or positive relative accommodation, PRA) and recovery,
- BCC at 11 inches (28 cm) with no prism,
- Base-in and base-out fusional vergence ranges at 16 inches (OEP test numbers 17 and 16).

The sequence in which Pratt did these tests and more information on how he did them can be found in Appendix 2.

ASPECTS OF PRATT'S NEAR TESTING PROCEDURES

For near cross cylinder testing, Pratt preferred a diagonal cross grid over a horizontal and vertical cross grid. He felt that accommodation and convergence changes were less likely to occur and that perceptual and psychological factors were less likely to affect results when the patient was comparing up-and-to-the-left and up-and-to-the-right lines rather than comparing up-and-down and across lines.[2] He marked the up-and-to-the-right lines with one dot and the up-and-to-the-left lines with two dots so that the patient could more easily respond by saying one or two. (see Figure 2.1) On cross cylinder testing, Pratt recorded the lens power where the patient judged the two sets of lines to be equally black and distinct, or if there was no equal response, he recorded the eighth of a diopter lens power between the two lens powers on either side of reversal.

On the Bausch & Lomb Greens' Refractor that Pratt used, the cross cylinder lenses used for the BCC test were the same as the lenses used for the Jackson cross cylinder test for astigmatism. Cross cylinder lenses of different powers were available and could easily be exchanged in the refractor. Pratt used a cross cylinder with +/-0.50 D power for his near testing. Pratt did not reduce illumination for his near cross cylinder testing as on the OEP 14A and 14B tests and as is usually taught today.

The nearpoint test card designed by Pratt shown in Figure 2.1 was rounded on the bottom to reduce the likelihood that patients might attempt to fuse the diplopic edges of the card during dissociated phoria testing. Alternatively, Pratt sometimes used a card with a black background surrounding the central test target with black letters on white for dissociated phoria testing (his black background test target can be seen in Figure 2.2).

It may be noted in the list of tests above that Pratt used blur out as the endpoint on NRA testing rather than the first blur as is usually taught today. The rationale frequently given for the latter endpoint is so that lens changes do not go so far into the patient's depth of focus. Pratt may have preferred blur out because it may be more easily recognized by untrained observers.

STUDY ON THE EFFECT OF CROSS GRID ORIENTATION ON BCC RESULTS

In 1972, Pratt was the advisor for a fourth-year student research project which tested the effect of differences in the orientation of the cross grid pattern used in the binocular cross cylinder test. Black and Isaacson[3] did BCC tests with the cross cylinder minus cylinder axis at settings of 90, 180, 45, 135, 67, and 157 degrees. Cross grids were presented to the subjects with lines paralleling those orientations. The cross cylinder power was +/-0.50 D. The tests were done first with a plus pre-set starting point, with plus reduced to the test endpoint. The various grid orientations were presented in random order. Then the tests were repeated with a minus pre-set starting point and plus increased to the test endpoint. Grid orientations were also changed in a random order for the minus pre-set condition.

Thirty-nine optometry students served as subjects. Testing was done using a Bausch & Lomb Greens Refractor with the test targets set at 40 centimeters. Correlation coefficients of the results with 90/180 vs. 45/135, 90/180 vs. 67/157, and 45/135 vs. 67/157 were all $r = 0.97$ or $r = 0.98$ for both plus pre-set and minus pre-set conditions. Analysis of variance did not show a statistically significant difference in the test results between the three different orientations.

Although the numerical results of the study did not show an effect of grid orientation, Black and Isaacson noted that many of their subjects "subjectively reported that they had more difficulty in making a response when the target was oriented at the 90-180 position than when it was oriented at either of the two oblique meridians." They also observed from their viewpoint as examiners in this study and in the clinic that "a sizable portion [of persons] respond with less hesitation and greater sureness when the target is not oriented in the vertical-horizontal meridians." Black and Isaacson put forward two possible explanations for those results. First, such response patterns might be explained by an unconscious bias toward either horizontal or vertical because most of the objects in our world have vertical and horizontal features. Second, people might be less critical of horizontal/vertical differences because the great majority of cases of astigmatism have principal meridians close to horizontal and vertical.

Next, the monocular plus-to-blur-out test and the Pratt near cylinder test will be examined in more detail because it appears that they are somewhat unique and that they seem to have been originated by Pratt.

MONOCULAR PLUS TO BLUR OUT OR 21M TEST

For this test, the phoropter is set at the near PD, standard room illumination is used, and the nearpoint light is directed toward the near test target which contains a line of 20/20 reduced Snellen letters set at a distance of 16 inches (40 cm).[4] During the test, the patient is instructed to call out the letters in that line and to continue reading them quietly and then say "blur" when they become so blurry that none of them can be identified.

The test begins with the examiner occluding the left eye and adding plus over the right eye in 0.25 D steps. After the patient reports the blur, the examiner should wait a brief moment and ask, "Is it still blurred?" If not, more plus is added to a complete blur out. When that blur out is reached, the examiner adds 0.50 D more plus and starts reducing plus and instructs the patient, "When you can again read all the letters in that line, say 'now.'" Plus is reduced in 0.25 D steps and the point at which the patient says "now" indicates a recovery lens.

Then the right eye is occluded and the procedure is repeated for the left eye. Next, the right eye and left eye are tested separately, in the same way, a second time and then again a third time. The second and third phases are started with the recovery lens from the previous phase in place. The blur out and recovery lenses will frequently be more plus on the second and third phases than on the previous phase, indicating a greater relaxation of accommodation. The repetitions in the second and third phases are especially useful for patients with hyperopia, but often not needed for patients with myopia.

The blur out and recovery on the third phase are the endpoints that are recorded for the test. Because the test is done monocularly, convergence does not affect those endpoints.

Anecdotally, Pacific University graduates who learned this test in school have found it to be useful in determining the binocular balance. It does not appear that any published studies have been done comparing the anisometropia found with it to the amount found with other standard binocular balance tests.

The monocular plus-to-blur-out is usually about 3.25 D more plus and the recovery about 2.75 D more plus than the distance subjective refraction.[5]

PRATT NEAR CYLINDER TEST FOR ASTIGMATISM

Pratt found little difference between astigmatism measured at near and astigmatism measured at far, but he preferred testing at near because he found it to be quicker and easier. In addition, he felt that results were less affected at near than at far if the ocular refractive system was out of conjugacy with the test target.[6] He also felt that the near cylinder test was particularly good for presbyopic patients.[6]

The Pratt near cylinder test is started with the recovery lens from the monocular plus-to-blur-out (21m) test. If a high cylinder is found on keratometry, the Javal's rule estimated cylinder can be placed in the phoropter. The test distance is 16 inches (40 cm). Illumination is the same as on the 21m test. Two test cards are required, one with a horizontal/vertical cross grid and one with an oblique 45 degree/135 degree cross grid (or one card with one of the cross grids on one side and the other cross grid on the other side, see Figure 2.1). It is helpful to mount the two cards back to back in the nearpoint test card holder (or the one card with grids on either side by itself in the test card holder) so that it is easy to flip from one grid to the other. The test is done monocularly and started with the patient viewing the horizontal/vertical cross grid. It is conducted following these steps[7]:

1) The patient is asked whether the lines going up and down or the lines going across are blacker and more distinct. If the patient's answer is up and down, the minus cylinder axis in the phoropter is set at 180 degrees. If the answer is across, the minus cylinder axis is set at 90 degrees.

2) The patient is instructed to report which set of lines is blacker and more distinct after each lens change. The examiner adds minus cylinder power until the patient says the other set of lines becomes blacker and more distinct (reversal). After each 0.50 D addition of minus cylinder, 0.25 D plus sphere should be added to maintain the spherical equivalent.

3) After reversal, the oblique cross grid is put in place. Ask the patient which set of lines is blacker and more distinct, the ones going up and to the left or the ones going up and to the right. If the patient says up and to the right, the cylinder axis is rotated slowly toward 45 degrees

until the patient says the lines going up and to the left become blacker and more distinct (reversal). If the patient says the lines up and to the left in response to the initial question with the oblique cross grid, the cylinder axis is rotated toward 135 degrees until reversal.
4) When reversal is obtained, rotate the cylinder axis back toward the initial position, and ask the patient to report when the two sets of lines are equally black and distinct.
5) Now have the patient again view the horizontal/vertical cross grid. If the two sets of lines are equally black and distinct, the test is complete. If the set of lines that most closely parallels the cylinder axis is blacker and more distinct, reduce the minus cylinder power in 0.25 D steps equality is reached. If the opposite set of lines is blacker and more distinct, minus cylinder power is increased in 0.25 D steps until equality is reached. (For each 0.50 D change in cylinder power, sphere power is changed 0.25 D to maintain the spherical equivalent) When equality is reached, the test is complete and the cylinder power and axis in the phoropter is the correcting cylinder.

If the keratometer or a previous refraction indicates oblique principal meridians, the test can be started (steps 1 and 2 above) with the oblique cross grid, and then the horizontal/vertical cross grid can be used for axis determination (step 3 above).

STUDIES ON THE PRATT NEAR CYLINDER TEST

To date, at least three studies[8,9,10] have compared the results of the Pratt near cylinder test to other astigmatism tests, including the Jackson cross cylinder (JCC) test, considered to be the standard today. The examiners in each of these three studies were fourth-year optometry students.

Adams et al.[8] compared results on 134 eyes with the Pratt near cylinder test, JCC, and the four-ball cylinder test. Cylinder powers in the subjects ranged from 0.25 D to 4.50 D. The four ball cylinder test used one ball with vertical lines, one with horizontal lines, one with lines up and to the left, and one with lines up and to the right, thus being similar to the Pratt test but done at far with targets from a Bausch & Lomb projector. For analysis, they broke each cylinder down into its 90/180 and 45/135 components.

The average 90/180 differences were:

- 0.03 D (standard deviation of the differences = 0.26 D) between the Pratt test and the JCC,
- 0.003 D (SD = 0.33 D) between the Pratt test and the four-ball test,
- 0.05 D (SD = 0.33 D) between the JCC and four-ball test.

The average 45/135 differences were:

- 0.02 D (SD = 0.22 D) between the Pratt test and the JCC,
- 0.01 D (SD = 0.30 D) between the Pratt test and four-ball test,
- 0.03 D (SD = 34 D) between the JCC and the four-ball test.

Adams et al. concluded that the results were similar on the three tests.

Graf and Weaver[9] each did the following tests on both eyes of 20 first-year optometry students: Pratt near cylinder test, JCC test, and Preston test. The Preston test for astigmatism uses a sunburst pattern of radial lines 15 degrees apart, and was done at 40 cm with "procedural aspects... similar to the conventional clockdial test."

Because Graf and Weaver both examined each subject with all three tests, they had data for interexaminer repeatability, as well as for comparisons of the three tests. They found the following correlation coefficients when they compared the cylinder power obtained between the two examiners: Pratt test, $r = 0.87$; JCC, $r = 0.89$; Preston test, $r = 0.90$. Because the correlation coefficients were that high, they pooled their data together for comparisons of the three tests. The mean differences in the magnitude of the cylinder power were:

- Pratt – Preston, 0.11 D,
- Pratt – JCC, 0.05 D,
- JCC – Preston, 0.05 D.

Graf and Weaver's axis results were presented in three axis difference histograms showing the frequency of various levels of difference. One histogram showed the differences between examiners on each of three tests, another showed differences between the three tests for examiner #1, and the third showed differences between the three tests for examiner #2. In each histogram, the most common difference was less than 5 degrees, and the majority of differences were less than 10 degrees. As would be expected, axis differences between tests were less when cylinder powers were higher. For examiner #1, there were no axis differences greater than 30 degrees from one test to another in subjects with a cylinder power of 1.00 D or more. For examiner #2, there were no axis differences greater than 15 degrees for cylinder powers of 0.75 D or more. For examiner #1, the number of eyes for which the axis difference was 10 degrees or less between tests was greatest for the Pratt and JCC comparison. For examiner #2, the number of eyes for which the axis difference was 10 degrees or less between tests was greatest for the Preston and JCC comparison.

The purpose of the Graf and Weaver study was to evaluate the Preston test and they concluded that it could be used in place of the JCC to measure subjective cylinder power and axis. Their data also showed that all three tests compared fairly well with each other.

In a study by Johnson et al.,[10] astigmatism test results were compared for three tests on 40 subjects who were between the ages of 18 and 40 years and had at least 0.50 D of astigmatism. All three tests were done by two examiners. The three tests were: (1) the Jackson cross cylinder test (JCC) done in the standard manner with one eye occluded, (2) The JCC test done with the binocular refraction procedure known as the Humphriss immediate contrast (HIC) method in which the eye not being tested is blurred by +0.75 D to induce foveal suppression,[11] and (3) the Pratt near cylinder test.

Because both examiners did all three tests on all subjects in the Johnson et al. study, the interexaminer repeatabilities for each test could be assessed. The mean differences in cylinder power between examiners were: JCC, 0.08 D (standard deviation of the differences = 0.35 D); HIC, 0.11 D (SD = 0.20 D); and Pratt, 0.10 D (SD = 0.36 D). The authors concluded that all three tests showed good repeatability.

In the Johnson et al. study, the differences in cylinder power between tests were:

- The JCC cylinder power minus the HIC cylinder power averaged 0 D (SD = 0.20 D) for examiner #1 and -0.03 D (SD = 0.17 D) for examiner #2.
- The mean JCC minus Pratt power difference was -0.08 D (SD = 0.28 D) for examiner #1 and -0.10 D (SD = 0.20 D) for examiner #2.
- The HIC minus Pratt power difference averaged -0.08 D (SD = 0.25 D) for examiner #1 and -0.08 D (SD = 0.22 D) for examiner #2.

Johnson et al. also found small mean differences in axis which were not statistically significant by paired t-test in each of the comparisons of tests (JCC vs. HIC, JCC vs, Pratt, and Pratt vs. HIC).[12] They concluded that "Pratt and HIC techniques can be used as optional methods for the JCC in determining the cylindrical portion of a spectacle prescription."[10]

A potentially important difference of the Pratt near cylinder test from the JCC test is that the Pratt test is performed at near. Some investigators have suggested that there may be individuals who manifest changes in astigmatism associated with changes in accommodation.[13,14,15] However, the three studies reviewed above show a reasonable agreement between the Pratt near cylinder test and the JCC test.

Like the JCC test, the Pratt near cylinder test is performed monocularly. It has been noted that patients with cyclophorias could have differences in cylinder axis going from monocular to binocular conditions, a factor which could become important if the amount of cylinder were high enough.[16,17] A study by Blake et al.[18] addressed the matter of the Pratt near cylinder test being a monocular test by comparing results obtained with it on both eyes of 52 subjects under monocular and binocular conditions. Subjects were 18 to 40 years of age. The same test targets and procedures were used for testing under monocular and binocular conditions, except that for the monocular condition, the eye not being tested was occluded, and that for the binocular condition, the eye not being tested was blurred by +0.75 D. A circle was drawn around each of the cross grid patterns to help maintain peripheral fusion for the binocular condition.

Differences in cylinder power between monocular and binocular conditions were 0 in 63% of eyes, 0.25 D in 33% of eyes, and 0.50 D in 4% of eyes. Differences in cylinder axis were 5 degrees or less in 87% of eyes overall and 12 of 15 (80%) of eyes with more than 1.00 D of astigmatism. There was one eye out of four with astigmatism greater than 2.00 D that had an axis difference of more than 5 degrees. Blake et al. suggested that for cylinder powers of 2.00 D or less, differences in cylinder axis between monocular and binocular conditions were clinically insignificant. They did not mention whether they had checked for cyclophoria in their subjects.

FARPOINT REFRACTIVE TESTS PERFORMED BY PRATT

For many years in his practice, Pratt performed a series of refractive tests at farpoint.[19] For farpoint testing he used a Bausch & Lomb Clason projector or a Bausch & Lomb Compact Acuity projector[20,21] with the projector screen 5 meters from the patient. Included among the tests performed at farpoint by Pratt were:

- Red-green test,
- Cross cylinder at distance,
- von Graefe dissociated phoria through the distance refraction,
- Maximum plus to 2/3 of the 20/20 letters and maximum plus to best visual acuity (similar to OEP test numbers 7 and 7A),
- Base-in and base-out fusional vergence ranges (OEP test numbers 11, 9, and 10).

For the red-green test, Pratt recorded the spherical lens powers through which the patient judged letters (20/40 black letters, two on the red background and two on the green background) to have "equal blackness and distinctness, or a reversal of the direction of inequality" on the red and green backgrounds.[19] In the case of reversal, he recorded the eighth of a diopter value between the lens powers before and after reversal.

After the red-green test, Pratt did a cross cylinder test at distance. He recorded the spherical lens powers through which the patient reported "equal blackness and distinctness, or a reversal of the direction of inequality" of projected oblique cross grid lines. In the case of reversal, he recorded the eighth of a diopter value between the lens powers on either side of reversal. The distance cross cylinder target consisted of eight black lines parallel to one axis of a cross cylinder and eight black lines parallel to the other axis of the cross cylinder. The cross cylinder power was +/- 0.50 D. On both the red-green test and the distance cross cylinder test, Pratt started on the plus side.

Pratt also found the most plus power through which the patient correctly identified at least two-thirds of the letters in the 20/20 line (similar to the OEP #7 test), and the maximum plus to best visual acuity (similar to the OEP #7A test).

P-FACTOR

Pratt analyzed data from 560 examinations in his practice to calculate the mean differences between refractive tests. He found that:

- The maximum plus to best visual acuity (MPBVA) averaged 3.20 D less plus than the binocular plus-to-blur-out at 16 inches with 16 prism diopters base-in (standard deviation of the differences = 0.28 D).
- The MPBVA averaged 1.94 D less plus than the binocular cross cylinder at 16 inches with 16 prism diopters base-in (SD = 0.25 D).
- The MPBVA averaged 0.02 D more plus than the red-green test (SD = 0.23 D).
- The MPBVA averaged 0.23 D more plus than the cross cylinder at distance (SD = 0.18 D).
- The MPBVA averaged 0.55 D less plus than the most plus to at least two-thirds of the 20/20 line (SD = 0.23 D).

Then for individual examinations, Pratt used those averages as constants to add algebraically to the respective test results (Table 2.1). Next the values of each test result plus the constant were averaged to get what Pratt called the P-factor.[19] (The term was suggested by a colleague during a Pacific University optometry faculty seminar[22])

Rounding the constants to the nearest 0.25 D, the calculation for the P-factor becomes:

$$\frac{(21\text{w}/16\text{BI} - 3.25) + (14\text{B w}/16\text{BI} - 2.00) + \text{Bichrome} + (\text{Far CC} + 0.25) + (\text{Blur-in} - 0.50)}{5}$$

Alternatively, the differences found between tests could be rounded to the nearest 0.25 D and used to predict the MPBVA or used as a check on the accuracy of the MPBVA (Table 2.1). The monocular plus-to-blur-out at 16 inches (21m test) was not in Pratt's original formulation of the P-factor, but it was later reported that the blur out on the 21m test was usually about 3.25 D more plus than the MPBVA and the recovery on the 21m test was usually about 2.75 D more plus than the MPBVA.[5]

The P-factor was viewed as a value for refractive error that was more reliable than a single test finding. It was thus seen as a reliable starting point for measuring accommodation and as a metric for studying longitudinal refractive error changes.[5,19]

Table 2.1. Values to be averaged for calculation of P-factor and which can used to help predict or check the accuracy of refraction.

Test	Algebraically add to enter in P-factor calculation (derived by Pratt)	Algebraically add for prediction or check of refraction
Plus to blur out at 16 inches with 16Δ BI	-3.20 D	-3.25 D
Cross cylinder at 16 inches with 16Δ BI	-1.94 D	-2.00 D
Red-green test at distance	+0.02 D	0
Cross cylinder at distance	+0.23 D	+0.25 D
Maximum plus to 2/3 of 20/20 letters	-0.55 D	-0.50 D
Monocular plus to blur out at 16 in. (21m)		-3.25 D
Monocular plus to blur out at 16 in. recovery		-2.75 D

DATA RELATING TO THE CALCULATION OF THE P-FACTOR – DATA FROM DAVIDSON AND MEYER

Data that can be used for replication of the constants derived by Pratt for the calculation of the P-factor or the prediction or verification of refraction results were taken from a 1973 Pacific University O.D. thesis by Patrick Davidson and William Meyer.[23] They performed most of the tests in the Pratt examination procedure. They tested 20 subjects who were between the ages of 10 and 32 years.

Differences were calculated of the OEP test number 7A minus the result of various tests for which data were available. The mean differences and the standard deviations of the differences are presented in Table 2.2. The means in Table 2.2 can be compared to the values in Table 2.1. The mean differences for the red-green, distance cross cylinder, and maximum plus to 20/20 minus VA are close to the constants calculated by Pratt for the P-factor.

Table 2.2. Summary statistics for the differences found by calculating the OEP 7A test result (maximum plus to best visual acuity) minus the finding of the given test for data from Davidson and Meyer.[23]

Test	N	Mean	Standard deviation
Red-green test at distance, right eye	19	-0.01 D	0.25 D
Red-green test at distance, left eye	19	-0.07 D	0.42 D
Cross cylinder at distance, right eye	17	+0.18 D	0.26 D
Cross cylinder at distance, left eye	17	+0.15 D	0.27 D
Monocular plus to blur out (21m), right eye	17	-3.42 D	0.41 D
Monocular plus to blur out (21m), left eye	17	-3.44 D	0.29 D
Monocular plus to blur out recovery, right eye	17	-2.96 D	0.33 D

| Monocular plus to blur out recovery, left eye | 17 | -2.96 D | 0.25 D |
| Maximum plus to 20/20 minus VA | 20 | -0.46 D | 0.23 D |

DATA RELATING TO THE CALCULATION OF THE P-FACTOR – PIKE STUDY

Additional data replicating the constants Pratt derived for his calculation of the P-factor come from a study involving the examination of 40 subjects.[24] Four of the subjects were presbyopic. The mean age of the subjects was 26.6 years, with a range of 21 to 56 years. Testing was done with a Bausch & Lomb Greens Refractor and 0.50 D cross cylinders, as advised by Pratt.

Four tests were done essentially as Pratt performed them: plus to blur out with 16 Δ BI at 40 cm, binocular cross cylinder with 16 Δ BI at 40 cm, red-green test at distance, and cross cylinder at distance. A fifth test, recorded somewhat differently from Pratt, was the maximum plus to a clear 20/20 at distance (as opposed to the two-thirds of the 20/20 line used by Pratt). Data from the right eyes of the subjects were used in the analysis.

The mean differences of the distance refraction minus the various test findings and the standard deviations of the differences are shown in Table 2.3. The mean differences are very close to the constants derived by Pratt for his P-factor for the plus-to-blur-out with 16 Δ BI at 40 cm, the binocular cross cylinder with 16 Δ BI at 40 cm, the red-green test at distance, and the cross cylinder at distance. There was approximately a quarter diopter difference between Pratt's constant for the maximum plus to 2/3 of 20/20 letters and difference for the maximum plus to a clear 20/20 in this study, as would be expected.

Table 2.3. Summary statistics for the differences found by calculating the distance subjective refraction result minus the finding of the given test for data from Pike.[24]

	Mean	Standard Deviation
Plus to blur out at 16 inches with 16Δ BI	-3.33 D	0.22 D
Cross cylinder at 16 inches with 16Δ BI	-2.02 D	0.30 D
Red-green test at distance	-0.01 D	0.16 D
Cross cylinder at distance	+0.24 D	0.17 D
Maximum plus to clear 20/20 at distance	-0.31 D	0.21 D

References

1. Lesser SK. Fundamentals of Procedure and Analysis in Optometric Examination, 3rd ed. Fort Worth, TX: S.K. Lesser, 1934:1-63.
2. Pratt CB. Lectures in Optometry 756 course, Advanced Optometric Case Analysis, Pacific University, October 30 and December 4, 1974.
3. Black SR, Isaacson GH. An investigation into the effects of axis orientation on the binocular cross cylinder. O.D. thesis, Pacific University, 1972.
4. #21m Test, Optometric Procedures III class handout, Pacific University, undated (circa 1971).
5. Calculation of the "P" Factor, Optometry 508 class handout, Pacific University, undated (circa 1971).
6. Pratt CB. Videotaped lecture, Sept. 10, 1971, Pacific University videotape VT68.
7. Near cylinder test, Optometric Procedures III class handout, Pacific University, undated (circa 1971).
8. Adams RL, Kadet TS, White DM. Comparative study of four-ball cylinder test, Jackson cross-cylinder test, and near cylinder test. J Am Optom Assoc 1966;37:547-549.
9. Graf LO, Weaver JC. A clinical comparison of three astigmatic tests. O.D. thesis, Pacific University, 1987.
10. Johnson BL, Edwards JS, Goss DA, Penisten DK, Fulk GW. A comparison of three subjective tests for astigmatism and their interexaminer reliabilities. J Am Optom

Assoc 1996;67:590-598.
11. Humphriss D. Binocular refraction. In: Edwards K, Llewellyn R, eds. Optometry. London: Butterworths, 1988:140-149.
12. Johnson BL, Edwards JS. A comparison of three tests for astigmatism and their interexaminer reliability. Optometry Project course (Optometry 6022) paper, Northeastern State University, 1993.
13. Bannon RE. A study of astigmatism at the near point with special reference to astigmatic accommodation. Am J Optom Arch Am Acad Optom 1946;23:53-75.
14. Nicholson SB, Garzia RP. Astigmatism at nearpoint: adventitious, purposeful, and environmental influences. J Am Optom Assoc 1988;59:936-941.
15. Garzia RP, Nicholson SB. Clinical aspects of accommodative influences on astigmatism. J Am Optom Assoc 1988;59:942-945.
16. Wick B, Ryan JB. Clinical aspects of cyclophoria: definition, diagnosis, therapy. J Am Optom Assoc 1982;53:987-995.
17. Rutstein RP, Eskridge JB. Effect of cyclodeviations on the axis of astigmatism (for patients with superior oblique paresis). Optom Vis Sci 1990;67:80-83.
18. Blake HA, Richardson JA, Shirk WW. A study to compare two methods of near astigmatism testing. O.D. thesis, Pacific University, 1972.
19. Pratt CB. A basic unit applicable to myopic and non-myopic individuals, typescript, prepared for paper presented at American Academy of Optometry meeting in Houston, Texas, December 8, 1956.
20. Bausch & Lomb Ophthalmic Reference Book. Rochester, NY: Bausch & Lomb, 1948:237-267.
21. Goss DA. Historical note on distance test charts and projectors. Hindsight: J Optom Hist 2014;45:53-58.
22. Roberts J, Roberts JR, Haynes HM. As they see Carol Pratt. Oregon Optometrist. Nov.-Dec., 1966:5-6.
23. Davidson PE, Meyer WR. An interpretation of Pratt analytical techniques and comparison of near-point therapy to that of O.E.P. O.D. thesis, Pacific University, 1973.
24. Pike SE. A study of the p-value method of distance refraction estimation and the predictability of the distance refraction from two selected near tests. Pacific University symposium paper, April, 1976.

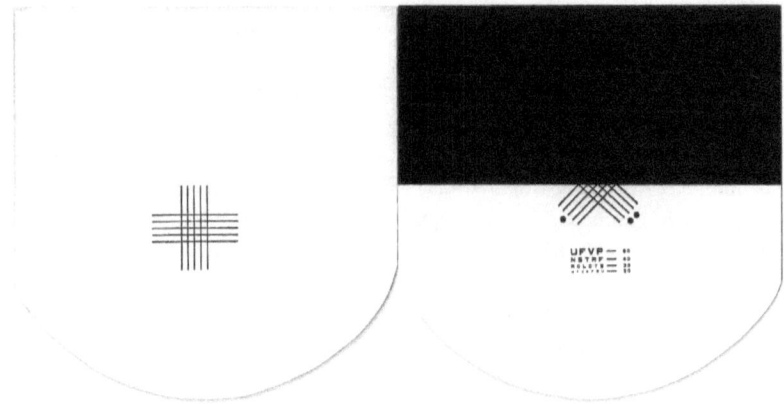

Figure 2.1. An example of the two sides of a nearpoint test card Pratt used for various tests. The two cross grids can be used in the Pratt near cylinder test for astigmatism and the oblique cross grid can also be used for cross cylinder tests. The bottom of the card is rounded to reduce the likelihood of the patient unconsciously trying to fuse the sides of the card during von Graefe dissociated phoria testing. (Photo taken by Scott Pike)

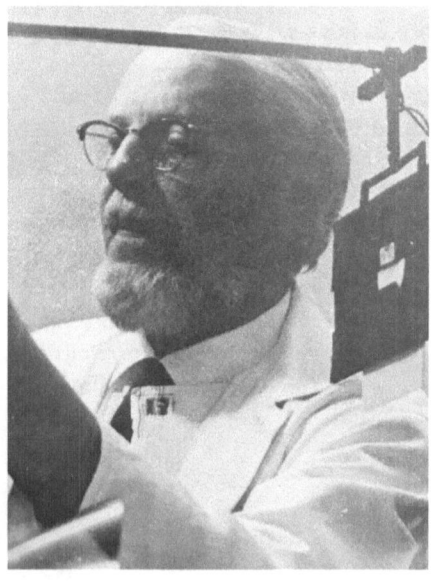

Figure 2.2. Pratt doing near testing. It may be noticed that there is a black surround around the central nearpoint target on the near test card. (Photo from Pacific University Yearbook, 1971, page 19)

Chapter 3

Pratt's Accommodation and Convergence Analysis System

Pratt used the tests he conducted at nearpoint (described in chapter 2) in the system he developed for analysis of accommodation and convergence function. He plotted the results of those tests on a graph with accommodation in diopters (D) on the x-axis and convergence in meter angles (MA) on the y-axis.[1,2] Accommodative stimulus in diopters is equal to the reciprocal of the viewing distance in meters for a patient viewing through the maximum plus to best visual acuity (MPBVA). Similarly, convergence stimulus in MA is equal to the reciprocal of the viewing distance in meters when the patient is not viewing through prism. Prism diopters can be converted into MA by dividing the number of prism diopters by the interpupillary distance (PD) in centimeters. Convergence stimulus in prism diopters is dependent in part on the PD, but convergence stimulus in MA is not, thus eliminating the effect of increasing PD with growth.

Accommodative stimulus for 40 cm (about 16 inches) for a patient viewing through Pratt's P-factor or through the MPBVA and no prism is 2.50 D. The convergence stimulus for an object at 40 cm, not viewed through any prism is 2.5 MA. The accommodation and convergence stimuli for objects viewed at various distances through P or the MPBVA and no prism is a 1:1 line across the graph (1 MA on the y-axis for every 1 D on the x-axis). This 1:1 stimulus line is called the demand line because it represents the demand on accommodation and convergence for different distances.

Plus lenses decrease the accommodative stimulus, and minus lenses increase the accommodative stimulus. Base-in prism decreases the convergence stimulus, and base-out prism increases the convergence stimulus. Thus, for example, for a patient viewing an object at 40 cm through a +1.00 D add, the accommodative stimulus would be 2.50 D − 1.00 D = 1.50 D. And for a patient with a 6 cm PD viewing an object at 40 cm through 6 Δ base-out, the convergence stimulus would be 2.5 MA + [6 Δ / (6 Δ/MA)] = 3.5 MA.

Normative data that Pratt derived are portrayed in Figure 3.1. The phoria and cross cylinder lines are approximately linear between 1 and 3 D, but frequently depart from linearity outside that range. The phoria and cross cylinder lines intersected at about 1 D on the demand line on average.

In Pratt's graph, the change in accommodation (Δx) divided by the change in convergence (Δy) on the cross cylinder lines represents the convergence accommodation to convergence (CA/C) ratio. The change in convergence (Δy) divided by the change in accommodation (Δx) on the phoria line represents the accommodative convergence to accommodation (AC/A) ratio.

For different patients, the slopes and lateral placements of the cross cylinder and phoria lines varied, but the phoria line tilted more to the right more than the cross cylinder line for all patients. The greater tilt to the right of the phoria line with the arrangement of axes Pratt used is consistent with the AC/A and CA/C findings of several studies.[3,4,5]

Pratt's normative data showed the cross cylinder line and the phoria line to be on either side of the demand line and approximately equidistant from it,[6] as shown in Figure 3.1. For a given patient, if the cross cylinder line was farther from the demand line than the phoria line, Pratt recommended prescribing a plus add for near that was equal in amount to the distance on the x-axis from the 2.50 D point on the demand line to the point midway between the phoria and cross cylinder lines at the level of 2.5 MA on the y-axis. These cases were typically convergence excess, basic esophoria, or accommodative insufficiency cases. They are considered accommodative lag cases in Pratt Analysis.[7]

If the phoria line was farther from the demand line than the cross cylinder line, Pratt recommended the prescription of base-in prism equal in power to the distance on the y-axis from the midpoint between the phoria line and the cross cylinder line to the point on the demand line at the 2.50 D level on the x-axis. These cases were typically convergence insufficiency or basic exophoria cases. They are considered convergence lag cases in Pratt Analysis.[7]

STUDY COMPARING PRATT NEARPOINT RECOMMENDATIONS TO THOSE OF OEP ANALYSIS

Patrick Davidson and William Meyer compared the prescription recommendations from Pratt Analysis and from Optometric Extension Program (OEP) Analysis for 20 subjects.[7] The subjects ranged in age from 10 to 32 years, with a mean age of 21.5 years. Seven of the 20 subjects had myopia of -1.75 to -5.25 D. Thirteen subjects had spherical equivalent refractive errors between -0.50 and +1.00 D.

Pratt Analysis recommended nearpoint plus adds for seven subjects. The powers of the plus adds ranged from +0.37 to +1.50 D, with a mean of +0.98 D. All seven of the subjects for whom plus adds were recommended had esophoria at near. Esophoria, moderate to high AC/A ratios, and binocular cross cylinder findings which were more plus than average resulted in the cross cylinder line being farther from the demand line than the phoria line. One of the subjects had significant esophoria at both distance and near, and the recommended prescription had both a +1.50 D near add and 1.5 prism diopters base-out prism.

Pratt Analysis recommended base-in prism for five subjects. The amount of base-in prism ranged from 0.75 to 1.5 prism diopters. These subjects had exophoria at near, low or moderate AC/A ratios, and binocular cross cylinder findings which were less plus than average. Their test findings resulted in the phoria line being farther from demand line than the cross cylinder line.

OEP Analysis does not recommend prism prescription. OEP Analysis recommended nearpoint plus adds for 14 of the 20 subjects in this study. OEP Analysis recommended plus adds for six of the seven subjects for whom plus adds were recommended by Pratt Analysis and for four of the five subjects for whom a base-in prism was recommended by Pratt Analysis. The powers of the plus adds recommended by OEP Analysis ranged from +0.50 to +1.25 D, with a +0.75 D add being recommended for 11 subjects.

MORE ON HOW PRATT PLOTTED HIS GRAPHS AND SOME EXAMPLES

Pratt plotted his graphs on graph paper, one square for each 0.25 D of accommodative stimulus on the horizontal axis and one square for each 0.25 MA of convergence on the vertical axis. When plotting convergence values on his graph, Pratt converted the power in the Risley prisms to the effective power in the presumed approximate plane of the centers of rotation of the eyes. Based on calculations for the vertex distance on his Bausch & Lomb Greens' Refractor, he plotted prism values which were 85% of the values shown on the Risley prisms.[8] He also converted lens values from the lens plane of the Refractor to the plane of the cornea for plotting accommodative findings.

When plotting binocular cross cylinder (14B) findings, the x-axis value was the accommodative stimulus for the test distance with subtraction of any amount of plus over the P-factor (or MPBVA) or addition of any amount of minus over the P-factor (or MPBVA). The y-axis value was the convergence stimulus for the test distance with subtraction of any amount of base-in prism or addition of any amount of base-out prism.

When plotting the unfused cross cylinder (14A) finding, the x-axis value was derived in the same way as for 14B tests. The y-axis value took into account the phoria taken through the 14A lenses (the 15A phoria). Thus the y-axis value was the convergence stimulus for the test distance with subtraction of any amount of exophoria in the 15A phoria or addition of any amount of esophoria in the 15A phoria.

When plotting phoria findings, the x-axis value was the accommodative stimulus for the test distance with subtraction of any amount of plus over the P-factor (or MPBVA) used during testing or addition of any amount of minus over the P-factor (or MPBVA). The y-axis value was the convergence stimulus for the test distance with subtraction of any amount of exophoria or addition of any amount of esophoria.

Figures 3.2 and 3.3 are examples of Pratt graphs plotted by the authors using data from the Davidson and Meyer thesis. Figure 3.2 presents the plot for a subject for whom Pratt recommended a plus add for near. The cross cylinder line is farther from the demand line than the phoria line due to higher than normal amount of plus on the binocular cross cylinder and esophoria at near.

Figure 3.3 is a graph for a subject for whom Pratt recommended a base-in prism. The phoria line is farther from the demand line than the cross cylinder line due to exophoria.

PRATT ANALYSIS PORTRAYED ON THE CONVENTIONAL ACCOMMODATION AND CONVERGENCE GRAPH

The clinical accommodation and convergence graph as it is taught at many optometry schools differs in format from that used by Pratt in his analysis. The conventional graph has convergence in prism diopters on the x-axis and accommodation in diopters on the y-axis.[9,10,11,12] We could potentially plot data like Pratt collected in his examination routine on a conventional clinical accommodation and convergence graph.[6]

For example, Figure 3.4 is a graph of the same data plotted in Figure 3.2. As in Figure 3.2, we can observe the cross cylinder line farther from the demand line than the phoria line. Figure 3.5 is a graph presenting the same test findings as in Figure 3.3, and like Figure 3.3, the phoria line is farther from the demand line than the cross cylinder line.

ACCOMMODATION AND CONVERGENCE FINDINGS IN PIKE STUDY

The accommodation and convergence graph data plotted in Figure 3.6 represent average findings from the examination of 40 subjects.[13] The age range of the subjects was 21 to 56 years (mean age, 26.6 years), with four of the subjects being presbyopic. Testing was done with a Bausch & Lomb Greens' Refractor. Data plotted include von Graefe dissociated phorias, cross cylinders, fusional vergence ranges, and relative accommodation findings.

It may be noted that the lines connecting the mean phoria points and the mean cross cylinder points appear much like the normative data plotted in Figure 3.1. The phoria and cross cylinder lines are on either side of the demand line and are roughly equidistant from it. The phoria and cross cylinder lines appear to intersect close to the one-meter point on the demand line. Breaks and recoveries are plotted for the base-in and base-out fusional vergence ranges. Blur out and recovery are plotted for negative relative accommodation testing. For positive relative accommodation, only the recovery was plotted because blur out was reached by larger steps in lens power rather than 0.25 D steps, as in keeping with Pratt's procedures in his later career, thus making the exact blur out endpoint uncertain.

COMPARING PRATT ANALYSIS RECOMMENDED PLUS ADDS TO SUBJECTIVELY PREFERRED PLUS ADDS

A study at Indiana University compared plus add powers recommended by various guidelines to the add power subjectively preferred by the study participants.[14] The 80 subjects in the study ranged in age from 18 to 30 years. The guidelines studied were various rules based on dynamic retinoscopy and normalization of the near dissociated phoria. Phorias were taken with the modified Thorington (tangent scale) method because of its high level of repeatability.

The study design made it possible to include evaluation of a modification of Pratt Analysis, with tangent scale dissociated phorias being used instead of von Graefe phorias, and one monocular estimation method dynamic retinoscopy measurement used instead of a series of cross cylinder tests. Otherwise, the modified Pratt Analysis in this study used the same basic graphical principle as Pratt's original analysis. Phorias were taken at 40 cm with plus adds for accommodative stimulus levels of 0.50 to 2.50 D in 0.25 D steps. A linear regression equation of phoria as a function of the accommodative stimulus was calculated to derive a phoria line. The midpoint between that regression line and the diopters of accommodative response on dynamic retinoscopy was found. The add which would yield an accommodative stimulus at the same dioptric level as that midpoint was taken to be the add power recommended by the modified Pratt Analysis (see Figure 3.7). Any negative value derived in that way was entered in the data analysis as zero, and any value over 2.00 D was entered in the data analysis as 2.00 D because 2.00 D was the highest add power used in the selection of preferred add.

For the selection of preferred add by the subjects, the examiners instructed the subjects to try sets of spectacles over their distance correction while reading from a magazine held at a measured distance of 40 cm and then to pick out the pair of spectacles that made the print easiest and most comfortable to read. The spectacles ranged in power from 0 to +2.00 D in 0.25 D steps.

The mean difference between the preferred add and the add from the modified Pratt Analysis was 0.04 D less plus with the Pratt guideline than with the preferred add. The standard deviation of the differences was 0.78 D. The low mean showed that on average the modified Pratt Analysis was very good at predicting the preferred add, but the relatively high standard deviation indicated that the predicted and preferred adds differed quite a bit for some subjects. Some variability may have come from the inclusion of asymptomatic subjects, thus perhaps making the selection of a preferred add by those subjects less obvious. Additional variability in the results may have come from how different subjects interpreted the instruction of using ease and comfort of reading as the criterion for selection of the preferred add.

CHANGES IN CROSS CYLINDER FINDINGS WITH AGE

Pratt used his patient data to investigate how the various cross cylinder tests he performed changed with age, particularly around the onset of presbyopia. He found little or no change in any of them from age 8 or 10 years up to age 35 or 37. Then the different cross cylinder tests started showing increases in plus (lower accommodative activity) at different ages: first the BCC at 11 inches, then a few years later the BCC from the minus side at 16 inches, then the BCC from the plus side at 16 inches (the standard BCC or 14B), and then lastly the unfused cross cylinder at 16 inches (14A).[15]

Similar results were found in a cross-sectional study by two students at Indiana University.[16] The mean findings on the standard BCC test on patients in the school optometry clinic showed minimal change from age 27 years to age 40, and then at 40 years, there was a steady increase in plus of about 0.1 D/yr to age 50.

Pratt also noted that his patient data showed the average minus to blur out at 16 inches (PRA or OEP #20) decreases in magnitude from about age 10 through young adulthood, reaching zero in the forties.[15]

OTHER MISCELLANEOUS PRATT RECOMMENDATIONS AND NOTES RELATING TO HIS STUDIES AND ANALYSIS OF ACCOMMODATION AND CONVERGENCE

- Pratt established norms for base-in and base-out fusional vergence ranges and for plus- and minus-to-blur-out at 16 inches (see Appendix 4), but the crux of his analysis system involved the cross cylinder and phoria findings and the graph as has been discussed. Pratt suggested that inhibitory findings should be taken before stimulatory findings because a stimulatory finding affects an inhibitory finding which would follow it. Therefore, base-in vergence ranges should be taken before base-out vergence ranges.[17] Studies have shown that base-out testing results in a greater fusional after-effect or vergence adaptation than base-in testing, thus agreeing with Pratt.[18,19,20] However, Pratt noted that some patients with high exophoria will relax on the base-in vergence and then not come in as much on the base-out vergence as they would have otherwise.[17] Based on the same principle of an inhibitory test before a stimulatory test, Pratt recommended doing plus to blur or blur out (negative relative accommodation, NRA) before the minus to blur or blur out (positive relative accommodation, PRA).
- Immediately after the break on lateral fusional vergence ranges, Pratt asked patients if one set of letters was higher than the other as a check to see if a vertical imbalance might be present.[17] When a vertical imbalance was confirmed by vertical phoria, Pratt preferred using the midpoint of the vertical vergence ranges for prescription of vertical prism.[21] Borish[22] also recommended using the midpoint of the vertical

vergence ranges to prescribe vertical prism.

- With sufficient practice and an appropriate form on which to plot findings, an accommodation and convergence graph can be completed quickly by hand with either Pratt coordinates or conventional coordinates. However, a common opinion is that it is cumbersome and time-consuming. That objection could be removed completely with a well-designed computer program that could interface with electronic health records. An example of a computer program that will complete an accommodation and convergence graph and do various analytical computations, including Pratt analysis, is one designed by Pacific University student Nathan Heilman for his O.D. thesis, with faculty member Scott Cooper as his advisor.[23]

References

1. Pratt CB. Videotaped lecture, Sept. 24, 1971, Pacific University videotape VT71.
2. Pratt CB. Lectures in Optometry 756 course, Advanced Optometric Case Analysis, Pacific University, November 6 and December 11, 1974.
3. Fincham EF, Walton J. The reciprocal actions of accommodation and convergence. J Physiol 1957;137:488-508.
4. Balsam MH, Fry GA. Convergence accommodation. Am J Optom Arch Am Acad Optom 1959;36:567-575.
5. Schor CM, Narayan V. Graphical analysis of prism adaptation, convergence accommodation and accommodation convergence. Am J Optom Physiol Opt 1982;59:774-784.
6. Goss DA. Pratt system of clinical analysis of accommodation and convergence. Optom Vis Sci 1989;66:805-806.
7. Davidson PS, Meyer WR. An interpretation of Pratt analytical techniques and comparison of near-point therapy to that of O.E.P. O.D. thesis, Pacific University, 1973.
8. Pratt CB. The variation in phorias with time after dissociation and magnitude of convergence. Am J Optom Arch Am Acad Optom 1962;39:257-263.
9. Pitts DG, Hofstetter HW. Demand-line graphing and the zone of clear single binocular vision. J Am Optom Assoc 1959;31:51-55.
10. Hofstetter HW. The graphical analysis of clinical optometric findings. In: Transactions of the International Ophthalmic Optical Congress, 1962:456-460.
11. Hofstetter HW. Graphical analysis. In: Schor CM, Ciuffreda KJ, eds. Vergence Eye

Movements: Basic and Clinical Aspects. Boston: Butterworths, 1983:439-464.
12. Goss DA. Ocular Accommodation, Convergence, and Fixation Disparity: Clinical Testing, Theory, and Analysis, 3rd ed. Santa Ana, CA: Optometric Extension Program Foundation, 2009:1-66.
13. Pike SE. A study of the p-value method of distance refraction estimation and the predictability of the distance refraction from two selected near tests. Pacific University symposium paper, April, 1976.
14. Goss DA, Rana S, Ramolia J. Accommodative response/stimulus by dynamic retinoscopy: near add guidelines. Optom Vis Sci 2012;89:1497-1506.
15. Pratt CB. Videotaped lecture, February 15, 1971, Pacific University videotapes VT43 and VT43a.
16. Gryschuk J, Meduna B. BCC progression in presbyopia, Epidemiology course project paper, Indiana University, 2013.
17. Pratt CB. Lecture in Optometry 756 course, Advanced Optometric Case Analysis, Pacific University, November 27, 1974.
18. Alpern M. The after effect of lateral duction testing on subsequent phoria measurements. Am J Optom Arch Am Acad Optom 1946;23:442-446.
19. Goss DA. Effect of test sequence on fusional vergence ranges. New Eng J Optom 1995;47:39-42.
20. Rosenfield M, Ciuffreda KJ, Ong E, Super S. Vergence adaptation and the order of clinical vergence range testing. Optom Vis Sci 1995;72:219-223.
21. Pratt CB. Lecture in Optometry 756 course, Advanced Optometric Case Analysis, Pacific University, December 11, 1974.
22. Borish IM. Clinical Refraction, 3rd ed. Chicago: Professional Press, 1970:872.
23. Heilman N. Computer based approach to graphical analysis: A Microsoft Excel application. O.D. thesis, Pacific University, 2003.

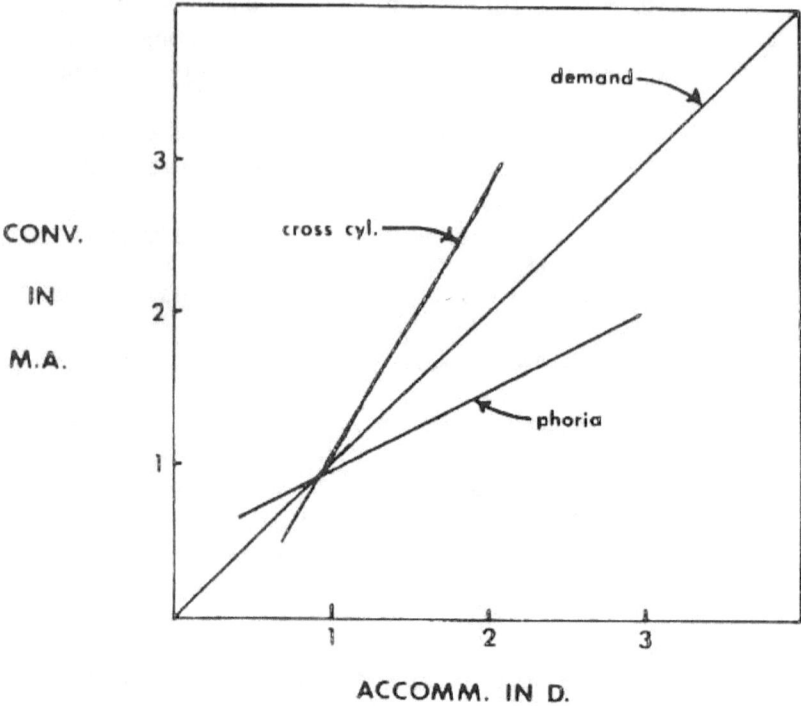

Figure 3.1. Normative data from Pratt with accommodation in diopters on the x-axis and convergence in meter angles on the y-axis. (Reprinted with permission from: Goss DA. Pratt System of Clinical Analysis of Accommodation and Convergence. Optom Vis Sci 1989;66:805-806. ©The American Academy of Optometry)

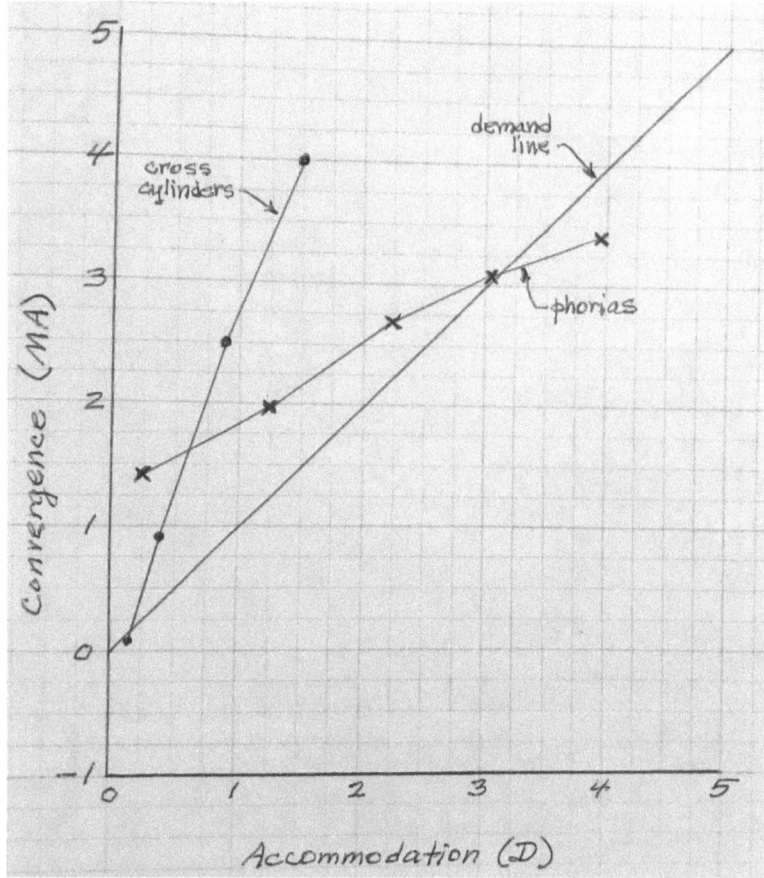

Figure 3.2. Pratt graph with corrections for vertex distance for a subject in the Davidson and Meyer thesis for whom Pratt recommended a plus add. (Graph drawn by the authors) Test findings were as follows:
- Binocular cross cylinder findings (14B) at 16 inches expressed as dioptric amount over the maximum plus to best visual acuity (MPBVA):
  With 16Δ base-in: +2.37 D
  With no prism: +1.62 D
  With 10Δ base-out: +1.00 D
- Unfused cross cylinder (14A) at 16 inches: +2.12 D over MPBVA
  Phoria at 16 inches with 14A lenses (15A): 11Δ exo
- Phorias at 16 inches with various lens adds over the MPBVA:
  With +2.25 D add: 6 Δ exo
  With +1.25 D add: 3.5 Δ exo
  With +0.25 D add: 1 Δ eso
  With -0.75 D add: 4 Δ eso
  With -1.75 D add: 6 Δ eso

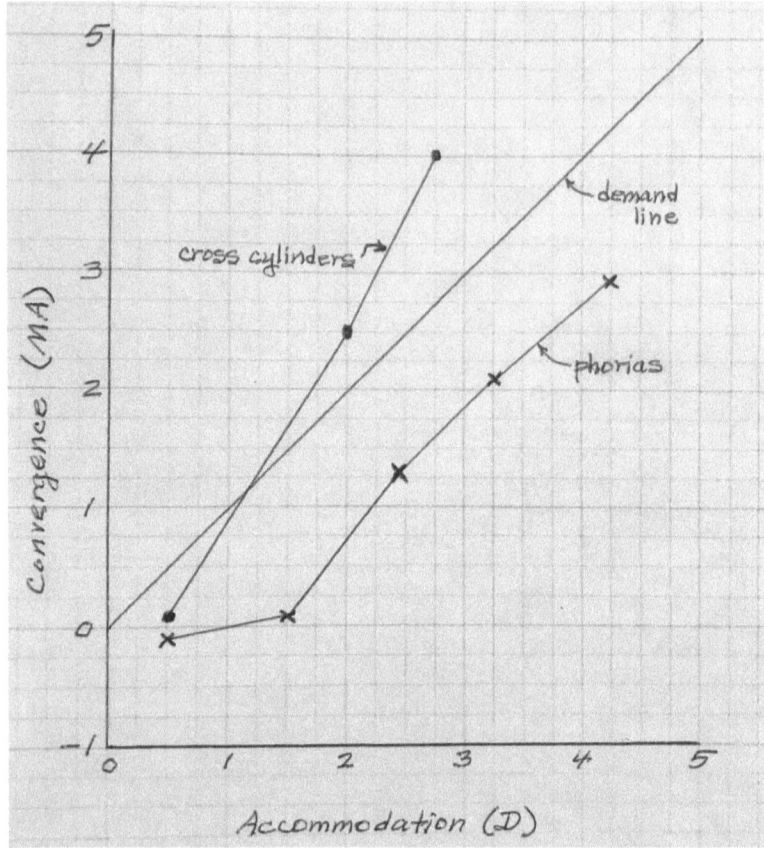

Figure 3.3. Pratt graph with corrections for vertex distance for a subject in the Davidson and Meyer thesis for whom Pratt recommended base-in prism. (Graph drawn by the authors) Test findings were as follows:
- Binocular cross cylinder findings (14B) at 16 inches expressed as dioptric amount over the maximum plus to best visual acuity (MPBVA):
  With 16Δ base-in: +2.00 D
  With no prism: +0.50 D
  With 10Δ base-out: -0.25 D
- Phorias at 16 inches with various lens adds over the MPBVA:
  With +2.00 D add: 18 Δ exo
  With +1.00 D add: 16 Δ exo
  With MPBVA: 8 Δ exo
  With -1.00 D add: 3 Δ exo
  With -2.00 D add: 3 Δ eso

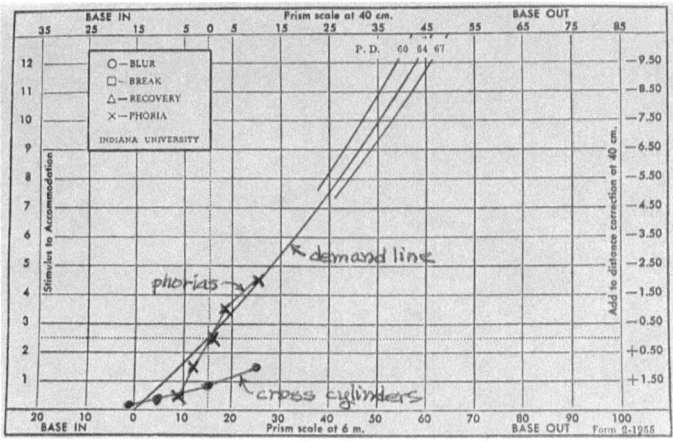

Figure 3.4. Conventional clinical accommodation and convergence graph with the same data as that portrayed in the Pratt graph in Figure 3.2. Here also the cross cylinder line is farther from the demand line than the phoria line, suggesting the prescription of a plus add. (Graph completed by the authors)

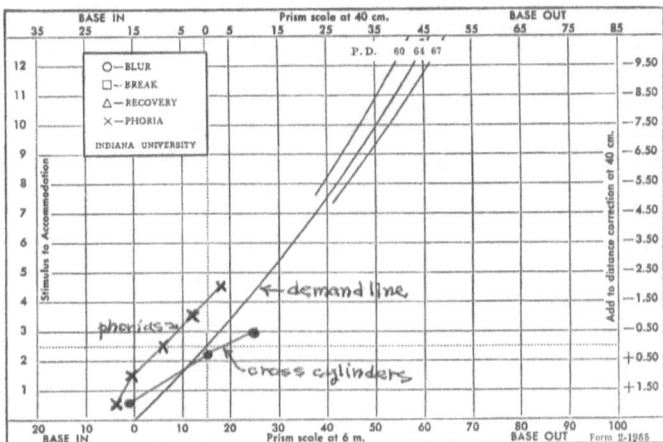

Figure 3.5. Conventional clinical accommodation and convergence graph with the same data as that portrayed in the Pratt graph in Figure 3.3. Here also the phoria line is farther from the demand line than the cross cylinder line, suggesting the prescription of base-in prism according to Pratt. (Graph completed by the authors)

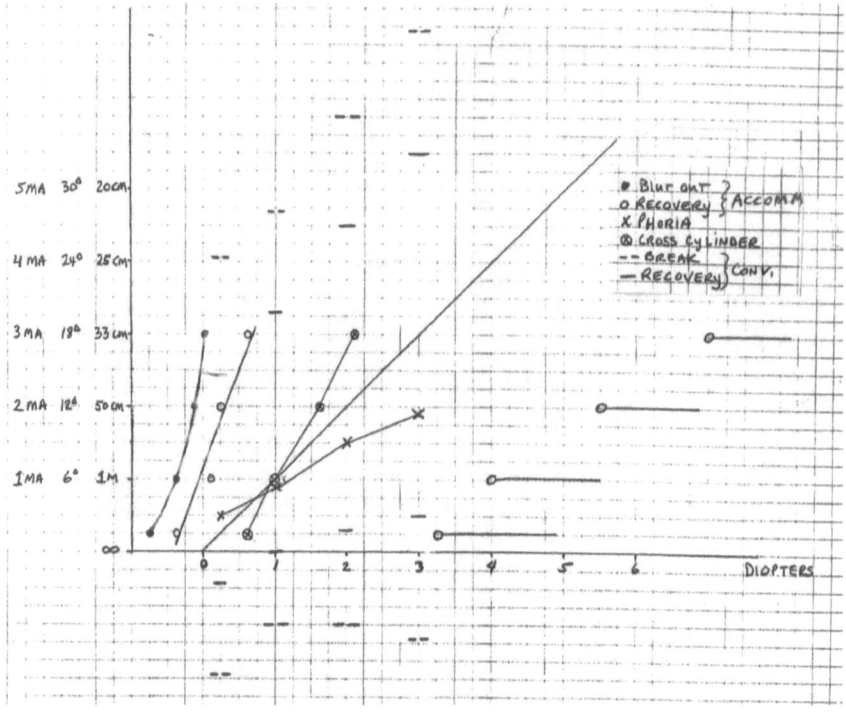

Figure 3.6. Mean data for phorias, cross cylinders, fusional vergence ranges, and relative accommodation for a group of 40 subjects from a study by Pike.[13] Accommodation in diopters is on the x-axis. Convergence in meter angles, prism diopters for an assumed 60 mm PD, and distance is on the y-axis. It may be noted that the phoria and cross cylinder lines appear to be very close to the normative data plotted in Figure 3.1, with an intersection close to the one meter point on the demand line. (Graph plotted by Scott Pike)

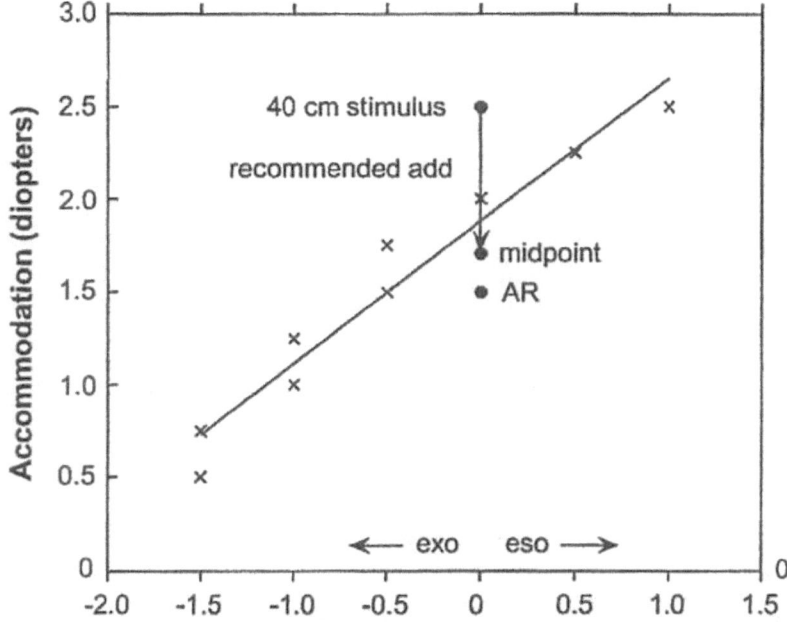

Figure 3.7. Illustration for one subject of the derivation of add power in a modified Pratt analysis system in a study comparing guidelines for prescribing plus adds to the subjects' preferred add. Convergence in prism diopters relative to a 40 cm stimulus is on the x-axis, and accommodation in diopters is on the y-axis. The x symbols are modified Thorington dissociated phorias at various accommodative stimulus levels. Positive numbers on the x-axis represent esophoria and negative numbers on the x-axis represent exophoria. The diagonal line is a regression line for the phoria points. The AR point indicates the accommodative response from dynamic retinoscopy at an accommodative stimulus of 2.50 D. The point labeled midpoint is halfway between the phoria regression line and the AR point. The point labeled 40 cm stimulus represents accommodative and convergence stimuli for an object at 40 cm viewed through the distance refractive correction. The add recommended by this analysis is the distance on the y-axis between the 40 cm stimulus point and the midpoint. (Reprinted with permission from Goss DA, Rana S, Ramolia J. Accommodative Response/Stimulus by Dynamic Retinoscopy: Near Add Guidelines. Optom Vis Sci 2012;89:1497-1506. ©American Academy of Optometry 2012)

Chapter 4

Pratt's Research on Refractive Errors

Pratt used the P-factor findings he calculated from examinations conducted in his practice to study longitudinal changes in refractive error. Results of those studies and some of his other refractive error research findings were among the topics he presented in his lectures at Pacific University. It may be noted that many of his research findings from the mid-twentieth century have been confirmed in papers published decades later. Pratt also devised a method of aniseikonia testing that could be done with a phoropter.

MYOPIA PROGRESSION

Pratt found the most common age of onset of myopia in his practice population to be at about 8 years of age.[1] Earlier onset was associated with greater rates of progression and higher amounts of myopia developed by adulthood. His data showed a slightly greater average rate of childhood myopia progression in females, but progression generally over a greater number of years in males, so that the overall increase in myopia averaged about the same in males and females.

Pratt found that childhood myopia progression tended to stop around the middle teens in females, and a little later in males. Males sometimes had continuing, but slower, myopia progression into young adulthood, on occasion to as late as 35 years of age.[1] Pratt's findings are supported by published studies that also reported earlier cessation or slowing of childhood myopia progression in females than in males,[2] and a slightly higher rate of childhood myopia progression in females.[3] Published studies have also replicated his findings of greater progression rates and higher amount of myopia developed by adulthood associated with an earlier incidence in childhood,[4,5,6,7] and more males than females having some continuation of myopia progression into young adulthood.[8]

In one of his lectures, Pratt presented illustrative cases of myopia in childhood, using graphs of the amount of myopia as a function of age to show typical patterns of myopia progression.[9] Similar graphs for individual patients are shown in Figure 4.1. These individual plots can be seen to show increasing myopia to the mid to late teens when progression tends to slow down or stop.

Pratt observed that if examinations were conducted at intervals of one or two years or more, the plot of myopia vs. age is essentially linear over most of the period of time that the myopia is progressing. This has also been observed in other studies,[10] and it can be seen in the plots in Figure 4.1. However, Pratt noted that when examinations were conducted at more frequent intervals, plots departed from linearity in two ways.[11,12] First, myopia progression appeared to have short periods of acceleration and deceleration. Perhaps that is related to the reports that myopia progression is greater during months when school is in session than during months which include the summer vacation.[13,14,15,16] Second, myopia progression tended to slow down a little before stabilizing in the mid to late teens, also seen in some of the plots for individual patients in Figure 4.1. Pratt observed that myopia progression was an exponential function when there were enough data points. This has also been reported in later published studies.[17]

Pratt also produced graphs of the average amount of myopia using a large number of patients with at least two diopters of myopia from his practice. Those graphs, one for females and one for males, are shown in Figure 4.2. Patients were grouped by the amount of myopia. Points in the graph were calculated by establishing rates of progression between examinations, then determining changes over quarter-year intervals based on those rates, and then averaging the myopia for all patients in the corresponding group at those quarter-year age levels. Some of the trends that Pratt talked about, such as earlier slowing of childhood myopia progression in females and higher rates of progression in children with earlier onset of myopia, can be seen in those graphs. The transition from progression to stabilization is smoother in the group average plots in Figure 4.2 than in plots for individuals in Figure 4.1 due to the variability in the ages at which different patients have slowing or cessation of their myopia progression.

Pratt did not take a stand on whether the primary cause of myopia was inheritance or environment. He did present an interesting case during a series of case presentations from his practice in one of his lectures.[9] He talked about a young man who had a typical pattern of childhood myopia progression followed by stabilization in his late teens. The period of stabilization lasted through years during which he was "a somewhat indifferent student in college." After college, he entered law school and experienced additional myopia progression. Pratt noted that the young man "had to bear down in his studies in law school," but stated that whether that was causative of renewed myopia progression was uncertain. His myopia progression in law school was at a lower rate than in childhood, as is typical of most cases of young adulthood myopia progression.

REFRACTIVE CHANGES AFTER 40 YEARS OF AGE

Pratt reported that in the absence of age-related cataracts, refractive changes after the age of 40 are somewhat different in hyperopic and myopic patients. Hyperopic patients increased in hyperopia by about 1.25 D in the 21 years from 49 years of age to 70 years of age.[18] His keratometer data suggested that about one-third of that increase in hyperopia could be accounted for by flattening of the cornea.[18]

Pratt found that many myopic patients became more myopic in their 40s and then start decreasing in myopia around 52 or 53 years.[12] Consistent with those findings, Grosvenor and Skeates found shifts toward hyperopia to be more common in hyperopic patients than in myopic patients, and shifts toward myopia more common among myopic patients than among hyperopic patients after the age of 45 years.[19]

ASTIGMATISM

For his studies on astigmatism, Pratt broke each cylinder down into its horizontal/vertical and oblique components.[20] This can be illustrated by the graph in Figure 4.3, which he drew. The cylinder axis is represented on the x-axis. The curve labeled rectilinear indicates the magnitude of the 90 or 180 component of the cylinder. The curve labeled oblique indicates the magnitude of the 45 or 135 component of the cylinder.

Take a cylinder of -1.00 x 15 as an example. The rectilinear curve shows a y-axis value of about 0.86 corresponding to the x-axis value of 15. The oblique curve shows a y-axis value of about 0.50 corresponding to 15 on the x-axis. Therefore, a -1.00 x 15 cylinder can be broken down into components of -0.86 x 180 and -0.50 x 45. Another graph drawn by Pratt to show components of a cylinder is Figure 4.4.

Pratt found that for non-presbyopes, with-the-rule astigmatism (minus cylinder axis 180) was about twice as common as against-the-rule astigmatism (minus cylinder axis 90). He noted that about 90% of his patients had a 90 or 180 component of at least 0.25 D. He found the amount of oblique astigmatism in the population to be very little. He did find that the oblique components to be mirror images in the two eyes of an individual, so that a patient with a minus cylinder axis 45 component in one eye tended to have a minus cylinder axis 135 component in the other eye. This mirror-image nature of astigmatism has also been reported in the literature.[21]

Pratt found minimal change in the oblique component of astigmatism between the ages of 49 and 70 years. Over that age span he noted an increase in against-the-rule astigmatism, which has been reported in other studies.[22,23] Pratt's data showed the increase in against-the-rule astigmatism from 49 to 70 years to be about the same as the increase in hyperopia over that age

Pratt also broke keratometer cylinders down into their 90/180 and 45/135 components. He observed the against-the-rule increase in refractive error in presbyopic patients to be about the same as the against-the-rule increase in the keratometer cylinder.[18] Other studies have found that most of the change toward against-the-rule astigmatism in presbyopes could be accounted for by changes in corneal astigmatism.[23,24,25]

COMPARISON OF ACCOMMODATION AND CONVERGENCE IN MYOPIC AND NON-MYOPIC PATIENTS

Pratt compared the results of some of his nearpoint tests in 40 myopic and 31 non-myopic non-presbyopic patients examined in 1957. The following are the differences he found.[26]

- The unfused cross cylinder at 16 inches (OEP 14A) averaged 0.44 D more plus in the myopic group.
- The dissociated phoria through the 14A lenses (OEP 15A) averaged 2.5 Δ less exo in the myopic patients even though their 14A was more plus.
- The binocular cross cylinder at 16 inches (OEP 14B) with no prism averaged 0.31 D more plus in the myopic group.
- The binocular cross cylinder at 16 inches with 10 Δ base-out averaged 0.50 D more plus in the myopic patients.
- The minus to blur out at 16 inches (OEP test 20) averaged 0.50 D less

minus in the myopic group.
- Dissociated phorias through various add powers over the P value were more convergent in the myopic patients by about two to three prism diopters.
- The binocular cross cylinder at 11 inches averaged 0.50 D more plus in the myopic group.

Consistent with Pratt's findings, there have been many studies that have found reduced accommodative function and more convergent phorias in myopes compared to non-myopes.[27,28,29]

ANISEIKONIA

For many of Pratt's years in practice, aniseikonia was a topic that was being widely researched in optometry, and the most commonly used instrument for its measurement was the American Optical Office Model Space Eikonometer.[30,31,32] Pratt did not think that it was a good instrument, so he devised his own method for measuring aniseikonia.[33] He used his Greens' Refractor to find the lenses that provided what he referred to as the spatial balance of the two eyes. The difference between the two eyes in the lenses that yielded spatial balance was compared to the difference between the two eyes in the P-factors to calculate the percent magnification of the aniseikonia. The steps in the procedure and calculations Pratt used are described in Appendix 5.

Pratt found that about 80% of his patients had a measurable amount of aniseikonia, but clinically significant aniseikonia was much less common.[33] He observed that the clinical significance of aniseikonia was dependent not only on the amount of aniseikonia, but also on the patient's sensitivity, with patients who made sharp judgments on aniseikonia testing being more likely to be affected by aniseikonia. Pratt sometimes specified particular surface curvatures or thicknesses of spectacle lenses[34] or made slight adjustments in the lens prescription to alleviate symptoms of aniseikonia.

References

1. Pratt CB. Videotaped lecture, March 1, 1971, Pacific University videotape VT48.
2. Goss DA, Winkler RL. Progression of myopia in youth: Age of cessation. Am J Optom Physiol Opt 1983;60:651-658.
3. Goss DA, Cox VD. Trends in the change of clinical refractive error in myopes. J Am Optom Assoc 1985;56:608-613.
4. Septon RD. Myopia among optometry students. Am J Optom Physiol Opt 1984;61:745-751.
5. Mäntyjärvi MI. Predicting of myopia progression in school children. J Pediatr Ophthalmol Strab 1985;22:71-75.
6. Grosvenor T, Perrigin DM, Perrigin J, Maslovitz B. Houston Myopia Control Study: A randomized clinical trial. Part II. Final report by the patient care team. Am J Optom Physiol Opt 1987;64:482-498.
7. Goss DA. Variables related to the rate of childhood myopia progression. Optom Vis Sci 1990;67:631-636.
8. Goss DA, Erickson P, Cox VD. Prevalence and pattern of adult myopia progression in a general optometric practice population. Am J Optom Physiol Opt 1985;62:470-477.
9. Pratt CB. Videotaped lecture, March 8, 1971, Pacific University videotape VT50 (also transferred from videotape to DVD).
10. Goss DA. Linearity of refractive change with age in childhood myopia progression. Am J Optom Physiol Opt 1987;64:775-780.
11. Hawks RL, Crowell GD. A longitudinal study of the progression of myopia. O.D. thesis, Pacific University, 1965 (advisor, C. B. Pratt).
12. Pratt CB. Lecture in Optometry 756 course, Advanced Optometric Case Analysis, Pacific University, November 20, 1974.
13. Fulk GW, Cyert LA. Can bifocals slow myopia progression? J Am Optom Assoc 1996;67:749-754.
14. Goss DA, Rainey BB. Relation of childhood myopia progression to time of year. J Am Optom Assoc 1998;69:262-266.
15. Fulk GW, Cyert LA, Parker DA. Seasonal variation in myopia progression and ocular elongation. Optom Vis Sci 2002;79:46-51.
16. Donovan L, Sankaridurg P, Ho A, et al. Myopia progression in Chinese children is slower in summer than in winter. Optom Vis Sci 2012;89:1196-1202.
17. Thorn F, Gwiazda J, Held R. Myopia progression is specified by a double exponential growth function. Optom Vis Sci 2005;82:286-297.
18. Pratt CB. Videotaped lecture, February 22, 1971, Pacific University videotape VT45.
19. Grosvenor T, Skeates PD. Is there a hyperopic shift in myopic eyes during the pres-

byopic years? Ophthal Physiol Opt 1999;82:236-243.
20. Pratt CB. Videotaped lecture, September 10, 1971, Pacific University videotape VT68.
21. Guggenheim JA, Zayats T, Prashar A, To CH. Axes of astigmatism in fellow eyes show mirror rather than direct symmetry. Ophthal Physiol Opt 2008;28:327-333.
22. Hirsch MJ. Refractive changes with age. In: Hirsch MJ, Wick RE, eds. Vision of the Aging Patient: An Optometric Symposium. Philadelphia: Chilton, 1960:63-82.
23. Lyle WM. Astigmatism. In: Grosvenor T, Flom MC, eds. Refractive Anomalies: Research and Clinical Applications. Boston: Butterworth-Heinemann, 1991:146-173.
24. Baldwin WR, Mills D. A longitudinal study of corneal astigmatism and total astigmatism. Am J Optom Physiol Opt 1981;58:206-211.
25. Naeser K, Savini G, Bregnhøj JF. Age-related changes in with-the-rule and oblique corneal astigmatism. Acta Ophthalmologica 2018;96:600-606.
26. Pratt CB. Lecture in Optometry 756, Advanced Optometric Case Analysis, Pacific University, November 6, 1974.
27. Goss DA, Zhai H. Clinical and laboratory investigations of the relationship of accommodation and convergence function with refractive error: A literature review. Documenta Ophthalmologica 1994;86:349-380.
28. Ong E, Ciuffreda KJ. Accommodation, Nearwork and Myopia. Santa Ana, CA: Optometric Extension Program Foundation, 1997:18-75.
29. Rosenfield M. Accommodation and myopia. In: Rosenfield M, Gilmartin B, eds. Myopia and Nearwork. Oxford: Butterworth-Heinemann, 1998:91-116.
30. Bannon RE. Clinical Manual on Aniseikonia: A Lecture Series. Buffalo, NY: American Optical Instrument Division, 1954.
31. Bartlett JD. Anisometropia and aniseikonia. In: Amos JF, ed. Diagnosis and Management in Vision Care. Boston: Butterworths, 1987:173-202.
32. Kulp MAT, Raasch TW, Polasky M. Patients with anisometropia and aniseikonia. In: Benjamin WJ, ed. Borish's Clinical Refraction, 2nd ed. St. Louis, MO: Butterworth Heinemann Elsevier, 2006:1479-1508.
33. Pratt CB. Presentations and demonstrations in Aniseikonia Special Clinic, Pacific University, February-April, 1974.
34. Rayner AW. Aniseikonia and magnification in ophthalmic lenses: Problems and solutions. Am J Optom Arch Am Acad Optom 1966;43:617-632.

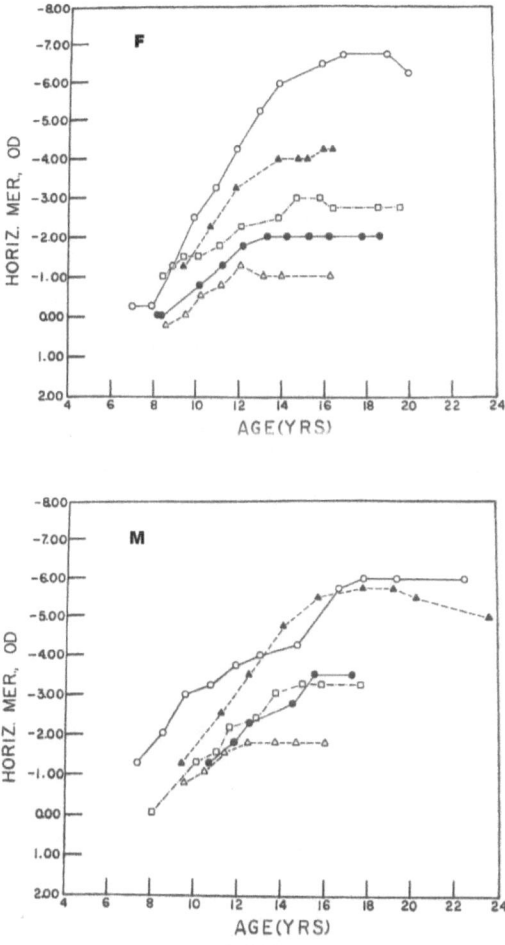

Figure 4.1. Typical patterns of childhood myopia progression followed by slowing or cessation of progression in the teens. Each set of common symbols represents the amount of myopia in the principal meridian nearest horizontal in the right eye for one individual. Pratt presented several cases of myopia progression in his lectures using graphs like these. The graph labeled F presents typical cases in females and the graph labeled M presents typical cases in males. (Reprinted with permission from: Goss DA, Winkler RL. Progression of Myopia in Youth: Age of Cessation. Am J Optom Physiol Opt 1983;60:651-658. ©The American Academy of Optometry 1983)

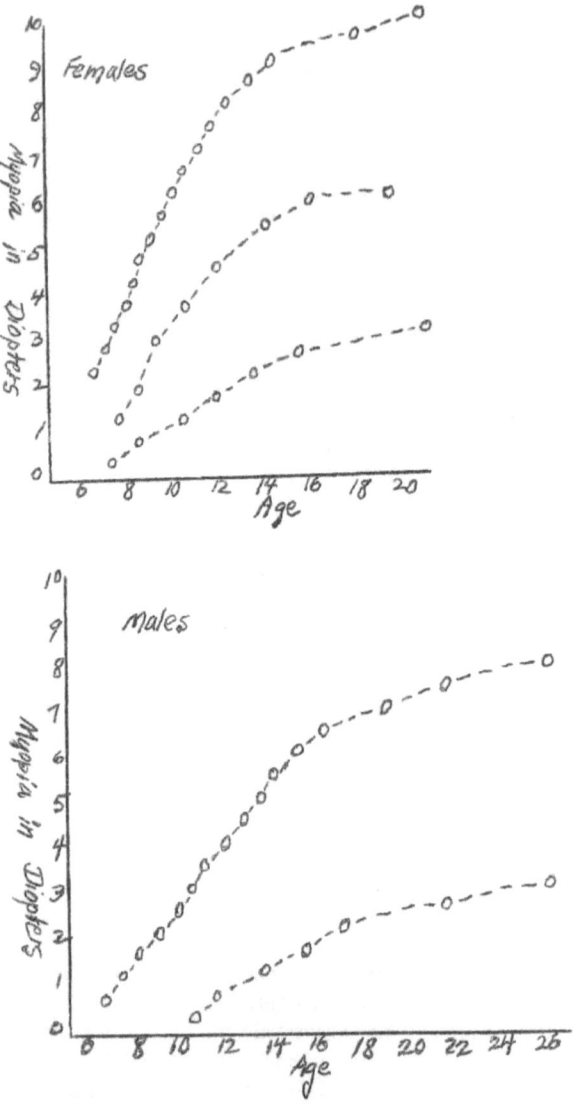

Figure 4.2. Graphs drawn by Pratt showing average amount of myopia as a function of age for groups of patients with more than two diopters of myopia. There are plots for groups of females with low, moderate, and high amounts of myopia in the upper graph. The lower graph shows plots for groups of males with low and high amounts of myopia. (From a class handout distributed by Pratt)

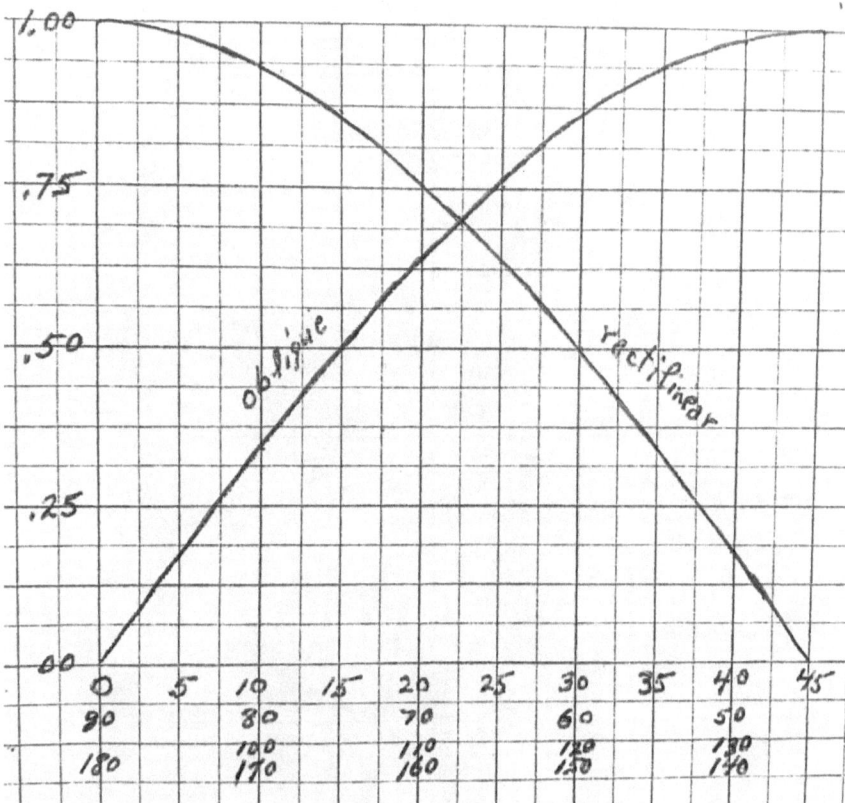

Figure 4.3. Graph drawn by Pratt showing breakdown of cylinders into 90/180 and 45/135 components. The x-axis indicates the cylinder axis. The y-axis indicates the percentages of power of the cylinder that are found in the 90 or 180 component (line labeled rectilinear) and in the 45 or 135 component (line labeled oblique). For example, for axes of 30, 60, 120, and 150, the rectilinear line passes through 0.50 on the y-axis scale and the oblique line passes through about 0.87. So a cylinder of -2.00 x 30 would have components of -1.00 x 180 and -1.75 x 45, and a cylinder of -2.00 x 120 would have components of -1.00 x 90 and -1.75 x 135. (From a handout distributed by Pratt)

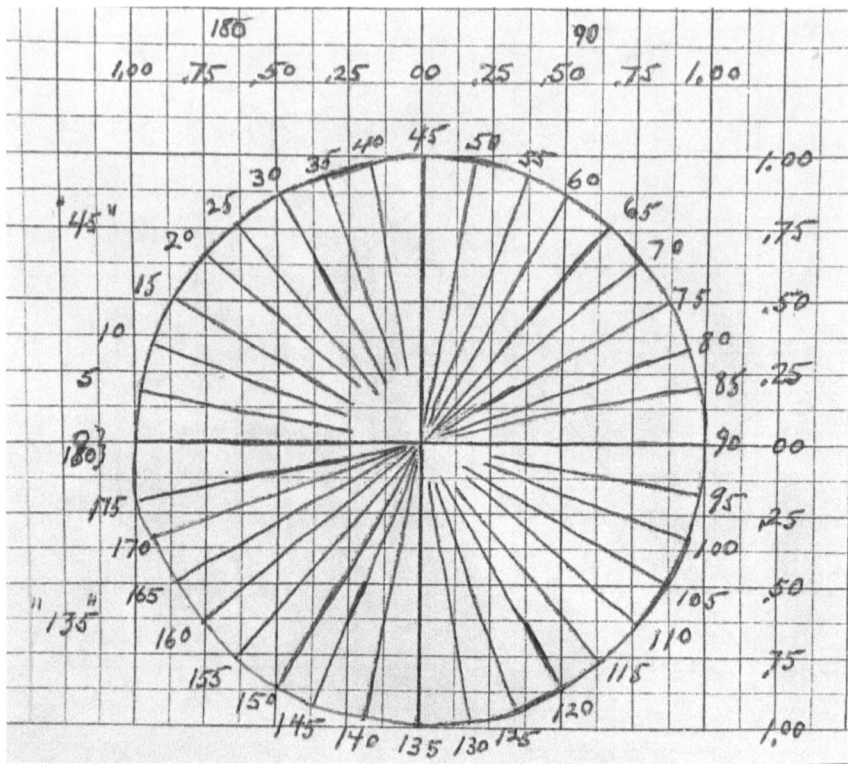

Figure 4.4. Another graph drawn by Pratt to show the breakdown of a cylinder into its 90/180 and oblique components. The upper scale shows cylinder power axis 180 to the left of zero and cylinder power axis 90 to the right of zero. The right-hand scale shows cylinder power axis 45 above zero and cylinder power axis 135 below zero. To find the powers of those components for a 1.00 D cylinder, locate the axis of the cylinder to be broken down on the circle and then see where that point on the circle falls on the two scales. For example, the components of -1.00 x 35 would be -0.34 x 180 and -0.94 x 45. (From a handout distributed by Pratt)

Chapter 5

Notes on Some Case Reports and Thesis Papers

Among the material that Pratt presented in his lectures were case reports from his practice. Another noteworthy aspect of Pratt's work is that he served as an advisor for many student thesis research projects. A selection of case reports and some thesis papers on which he was the advisor show his thinking on various clinical conditions and testing procedures.

CASE REPORT – USE OF A TINT IN ACCOMMODATIVE EXCESS

A case Pratt presented in one of his lectures illustrates his ability to think outside the box, making practical application of his knowledge of vision science and information he gained from some of his studies.[1] The case involved an 18-year-old college student who complained of slight headaches and occasional diplopia after studying. Pratt had examined him previously at 13 years of age, at which time he did not have any vision complaints. The patient's P-factor at 13 years was +0.62 D OU, and at 18 years, it was +0.37 D OU.

The patient's phorias at 18 years were within normal ranges, but binocular cross cylinder (BCC) findings were low. The BCC at 16 inches from the plus side was +0.37 D from the P-factor, compared to Pratt's norm of +0.87 D. The BCC at 16 inches from the minus side was -0.12 D compared to the norm of +0.37 D. The BCC with base-out prism was

-0.62 D compared to the norm of 0 D, and the BCC at 11 inches was -0.12 D compared to the Pratt norm of +0.87 D.

Pratt noted that the findings indicated an overactive accommodative system, a case referred to as minus projection in the OEP literature or as accommodative excess in other texts.[2,3] The common treatment for accommodative excess of vision therapy was not feasible in this case with the patient away at college. Pratt observed that another potential treatment might be base-in prism to inhibit convergence, and thereby reduce accommodation. He decided against prism because convergence was normal.

Pratt had conducted studies on cross cylinder tests at near under different levels of illumination, from very dim (just enough light to read letters) to very bright (standard room illumination plus full illumination with the near point light). His results showed that the brighter the illumination, the lower the cross cylinder findings were. In other words, increased illumination led to higher accommodation levels. For this patient, Pratt prescribed a tint to decrease accommodation.

The prescription was +0.25 D OU with a high optical density pink tint for reading and studying only. Two years later in 1952, when the patient returned for another examination, he reported that the glasses had alleviated his symptoms and he requested a replacement lens for one that he had broken. Pratt said that he had managed two other similar cases in this way and it showed that a case can often be approached in multiple ways.

After Pratt presented this case in his lecture, he mentioned an interesting conjecture.[1] He wondered whether illumination levels in school classrooms were too high. He speculated that illumination levels that were too high could drive accommodative levels and other physiological systems too high, perhaps contributing to the high reported prevalence of hyperactivity among students.

TWO CASES IN WHICH MYOPIA DECREASED IN YOUNG ADULTHOOD

As discussed in Chapter 4, Pratt observed that once myopia appeared in childhood, it increased until the mid to late teens and then remained stable for several years, or less commonly, it increased into young adulthood, albeit usually at a slower rate. Myopia can also have its onset in early adulthood, and then some progression at a fairly low rate. Pratt saw two cases in his career in which myopia decreased during young adulthood more than the +/-0.25 D fluctuations that could occur within the limits of repeatability of refraction. Both of these cases involved extreme psychological and emotional stress.[4]

Pratt prefaced the discussion of these two cases by saying that he thought that lecturers sometimes spend too much time talking about very unusual types of cases that students will never see in their careers. He stated that he presented these two cases because they demonstrated that there is more to the lives of patients than just a collection of test findings.

Pratt examined R. first when she was 13 years old, at which time she had low hyperopia. R. experienced very difficult socioeconomic conditions. Pratt examined her again at 19 years of age, by which time she had gone to work, as her father was deceased and she was the sole support for her mother and her siblings. She still had low hyperopia at that time. At 21 years old, her P-factors were about -0.37 D in each eye, and then at 26 years of age, her P-factors were about -0.50 D in the right eye and -0.87 D in the left eye.

R. was next seen when she was 28 years old. She said to Pratt that, "They tell me that I shot myself." R. had attempted suicide, shooting herself just above the right temple. The eye and the orbit were not injured but there was significant damage to the frontal lobe of the brain. Pratt found that her myopia had decreased and that she was now hyperopic in the right eye and only slightly myopic in the left eye. Cross cylinder findings that showed a high level of accommodative activity before the accidental frontal lobotomy now were fairly normal. Convergence findings that were previously normal now showed a high exophoria and the near base-out fusional vergence recovery was in the minus, needing base-in prism to recover. Pratt wondered whether the myopia R. had when she was in her early twenties was due to psychological stress, rather than changes in the structure of the eye.

The second patient, V., was the daughter of an optometrist with whom Pratt was well acquainted. Pratt first examined V. at 13 years of age. She had a typical childhood progression of myopia over the next few years. At 21 years of age, she was working as a bookkeeper, and her myopia was about -5.00 D in the right eye and -2.00 D in the left eye.

V.'s father had a fairly high amount of myopia and had a retinal detachment. Surgery for retinal detachment was unsuccessful and he became completely blind. V.'s family was very religious, and she saw her father's blindness as an act of God. Consequently she decided to enter a convent, thus experiencing a very different dietary, psychological, and emotional environment.

Pratt examined V. at 29 years of age while she was living in the convent. Her myopia had decreased to -4.00 D in the right eye and -0.75 D in the left eye. At that time, her cross cylinder findings showed less accommodative activity, particularly the unfused cross cylinder. Her convergence findings showed very little change, with the near dissociated phoria being normal at most examinations.

V. remained in the convent for eight years. She then attended college and entered the teaching profession. Pratt examined her after she started teaching and found that her myopia had increased back up to its previous levels. Pratt noted that the personality, lifestyle, and emotional changes in these two patients affected their visual systems, showing that the whole of the individual should be considered, not just test findings.

A SAMPLING OF O.D. THESES FOR WHICH PRATT SERVED AS ADVISOR

For many years, Pacific University College of Optometry required students in their final year of study to complete a thesis project. This project was referred to as the O.D. thesis. Students could work by themselves or in groups of up to four. Pratt was an advisor for many thesis papers on a variety of different topics during his career. A few of them will be discussed here.

A 1959 project by Harold W. Abare and suggested by Pratt, looked at how accommodation changed after reading through various lenses.[5] Twenty subjects read a paragraph of .62 M type (approximately 20/30) through various lens powers for 10 seconds after which the lens was removed and unfused cross cylinder tests were performed at regular intervals. The subjects ranged in age from 22 to 37 years. The lens powers through which the subjects read as measured from the P-factor were -3, -2, -1, 0, +1, and +2 D. Unfused cross cylinder tests were done at roughly 20-second intervals until three consecutive findings were the same or four consecutive findings varied over a range of 0.25 D. The minus adds initially decreased the cross cylinder findings (indicating an increase in accommodation) and the plus adds initially increased the cross cylinder results (indicating less accommodation), in amounts proportional to the power of the add. Then the cross cylinder findings decayed exponentially so that the average baseline level was usually reached by about two minutes. This study appears to have anticipated the extensive research done in the 1980s and 1990s on the timing of transient changes in accommodation after periods of reading and near work.[6]

A 1965 study by Gerald W. Bolokoski, Hugh R. Adair II, and Joseph J. Kvortek compared the interocular difference in corneal powers with the interocular difference in spherical equivalent refractive error.[7] Corneal power for each eye was based on the average of the powers in the principal meridians on keratometry. Refractive error was measured with standard optometric procedures (OEP 7A) to maximum plus to best visual acuity. A total of 102 subjects in the age range of 20 to 35 years were tested. Refractive errors ranged from -5.00 D to +2.00 D. Refractive error anisometropia ranged from 0 to 1.25 D. As the investigators expected, there was no correlation of interocular corneal power difference with refractive error anisometropia, even when subjects with less than 0.37 D of anisometropia were eliminated from the analysis. Studies with higher amounts of anisometropia have shown anisometropia to be most often due to interocular differences in axial length, with limited or no contribution from the cornea.[8,9]

Also in 1965, James C. Falconer and Gordon W. Postovit compared changes in corneal astigmatism to changes in refractive astigmatism in patients around the seventh decade of life.[10] Records were selected from the files of the Pacific University Optometry Clinic for persons close to 70 years of age at the time of the study who had examinations covering at least nine years. The recorded keratometer findings were used to calculate corneal powers in the 90 and 180 meridians. Subjective refraction data from the recorded OEP 7A findings were used to calculate refractive errors in the 90 and 180 meridians. The amounts of astigmatism were calculated from the differences between the 90 and 180 meridians. The average change in corneal astigmatism in 105 eyes over an average 11.2 year span (from an average of 58.9 years of age to 70.1 years of age) was 0.14 D toward against-the-rule based on keratometer power, or 0.15 D toward against-the-rule with correction for the presumed index of refraction of the cornea. The average change in spectacle plane refractive astigmatism over that same time was 0.16 D toward against-the-rule. The investigators concluded that the refractive error change toward against-the-rule in the selected age span was mostly due to corneal cylinder changes, a finding which has been reported in other studies.[11,12]

In another 1965 project, Ray Roy and Don Carkner studied the change in lateral dissociated phoria from straightforward gaze to 25 degrees downgaze.[13] The 25 degree downgaze position was set using an arc perimeter. To measure the phoria, a 10 Δ base-down dissociating prism was held over one eye, and a hand-held rotary prism was used over the other eye. Six phoria measurements were taken in each position. Subjects wore their habitual near prescription. For bifocal wearers, a trial lens with the same power as the bifocal add was held over the distance spectacle correction for testing in a straightforward position. There were 29 subjects in the 14 to 39 year age range, and 13 subjects in the 40 to 76 year age range. The phoria averaged 4.7 Δ exo in the straightforward position and 3.7 Δ exo in downgaze in the younger group of subjects. The phoria averaged 9.4 Δ exo in straightforward position and 6.7 Δ exo in downgaze in the older group. The difference in phoria as a function of gaze position was statistically significant for both age groups. Another study found slightly less exophoria at near in downgaze in non-presbyopic subjects.[14]

In 1969, Merci Jacobs and Earl Landry compared near von Graefe dissociated phorias with three different targets.[15] The targets were a reduced Snellen chart with letters ranging from 20/200 to 20/20, a cross grid with horizontal and vertical lines, and a single vertical column of letters of about 20/40 acuity level. Testing distance was 40 cm. Eighteen subjects participated in the study. Four phorias were performed with each target and with each of three lens powers in place (OEP 7A, 7A + 0.50 D, and 7A − 0.50 D). The mean phorias with 7A were: reduced Snellen, 3.9 Δ exo (SD, 3.1); cross grid, 3.5 Δ exo (SD, 4.1); and vertical column, 3.5 Δ exo (SD, 4.1). The mean phorias through 7A + 0.50 D were: reduced Snellen, 5.4 Δ exo (SD, 2.9); cross grid, 4.3 Δ exo (SD, 3.6); and vertical column, 4.9 Δ exo (SD, 4.0). The means with 7A − 0.50 D were: reduced Snellen, 2.3 Δ exo (SD, 4.2); cross grid, 2.1 Δ exo (SD, 4.9); and vertical column, 2.7 Δ exo (SD, 4.5). The differences were small, but slightly more exo was found with the reduced Snellen target. Standard deviations were somewhat lower with the reduced Snellen target. Subjects were asked after testing which target seemed to be the least confusing to align, and the predominant answer was the vertical line of letters.

M.S. THESES ON ACCOMMODATIVE RESPONSE MEASUREMENTS

In 1970 and 1971, Pratt was the advisor for three M.S. degree theses which compared various procedures for measuring accommodative response (AR). In each study, 30 subjects viewed a small block of 20/20 reduced Snellen letters. The accommodative stimulus (AS) was varied with +3 D, +2 D, +1 D, plano, -1 D, -2 D, and -3 D addition lenses. AR measured with a subjective method was compared to AR measured with an objective method in each study.

Bybee[16] compared AR with dynamic retinoscopy and with laser speckle refraction. The two methods showed close agreement in the AR mean values for each AS level and in the mean AR/AS slopes for each one diopter interval in AS.

Braun[17] compared AR using a Topcon Refractometer and a stigmatoscopic beam in a Badal optometer. The AR means with the two methods were not significantly different with the plano, -1 D, -2 D, and -3 D lenses, but showed mean differences of about 0.3 to 0.4 D for the +1 D, +2 D, and +3 D stimulus lenses.

Thomé[18] compared a bichrome method of measuring AR to the image size changes in the reflection from the anterior surface of the crystalline lens (third Purkinje image) with photographic ophthalmophakometry. The changes in AR with the bichrome method correlated well with the changes in the Purkinje image size change.

An overall trend that could be observed in the three studies was that the changes in AR for each 1 D step in lenses from plano to -3 D (AR/AS slope) were fairly close to the same (usually averaging about 0.6 to 0.8 D/D). Then from plano to +3 D, each 1 D interval in AS showed progressively less slope, with the slope between +2 D and +3 D being negligible. An AR/AS slope less than 1.0 D/D is consistent with the findings of many studies.[19]

References

1. Pratt CB. Videotaped lecture, March 29, 1971, Pacific University videotape VT75 (also transferred from videotape to DVD).
2. Manas L. Visual Analysis, 4th ed. Santa Ana, CA: Optometric Extension Program Foundation, 2009:38,332-333.
3. Scheiman M, Wick B. Clinical Management of Binocular Vision: Heterophoric, Accommodative, and Eye Movement Disorders, 3rd ed. Philadelphia: Lippincott Williams and Wilkins, 2008:363-371.
4. Pratt CB. Videotaped lecture, March 1, 1971, Pacific University videotape VT48a.
5. Abare HW. An experiment with cross cylinder findings at 16". O.D. thesis, Pacific University, 1959.
6. Ong E, Ciuffreda KJ. Accommodation, Nearwork, and Myopia. Santa Ana, CA: Optometric Extension Program Foundation, 1997:55-64,97-127.
7. Bolokoski GW, Adair HR II, Kvortek JJ. The correlation of the gross ophthalmometer anisometropia with the best far point acuity lens (O.E.P. #7A) anisometropia. O.D. thesis, Pacific University, 1965.
8. Sorsby A, Leary GA, Richards MJ. The optical components in anisometropia. Vision Res 1962;2:43051.
9. Laird IK. Anisometropia. In: Grosvenor T, Flom MC, eds. Refractive Anomalies: Research and Clinical Applications. Boston: Butterworth-Heinemann, 1991:174-198.
10. Falconer JC, Postovit GW. The relationship of the change of corneal power to the change in total refractive power of the eye with age. O.D. thesis, Pacific University, 1965.
11. Baldwin WR, Mills D. A longitudinal study of corneal astigmatism and total astigmatism. Am J Optom Physiol Opt 1981;58:206-211.
12. Lyle WM. Astigmatism. In: Grosvenor T, Flom MC, eds. Refractive Anomalies: Research and Clinical Applications. Boston: Butterworth-Heinemann, 1991:146-173.
13. Roy R, Carkner D. The relationship of the near phoria in the reading level and in the standard horizontal position. O.D. thesis, Pacific University, 1965.
14. Goss DA, Penisten DK, Pitts KK, Burns DA. Repeatability of prism dissociation and tangent screen near heterophoria measurements in straightforward gaze and downgaze. In: McCoun J, Reeves L, eds. Binocular Vision: Development, Depth Perception and Disorders. New York: Nova Science, 2010:155-160.
15. Jacobs MA, Landry EJ. Phoric measurements at near with three different target designs. O.D. thesis, Pacific University, 1969.
16. Bybee DA. A comparison of a subjective and an objective method of measuring accommodation using laser reflection and dynamic retinoscopy respectively. M.S. thesis, Pacific University, 1970.
17. Braun EG. Accommodative responses compared with objective refractometer and a subjective stigmatoscopic response. M.S. thesis, Pacific University, 1971.

18. Thomé CD. A comparative study of a subjective method and objective method of measuring accommodation utilizing a bichrome technique and photographic ophthalmophakometry. M.S. thesis, 1971.
19. Ciuffreda KJ, Kenyon RV. Accommodative vergence and accommodation in normals, amblyopes, and strabismics. In: Schor CM, Ciuffreda KJ, eds. Vergence Eye Movements: Basic and Clinical Aspects. Boston: Butterworths, 1983:101-173.

Chapter 6

Stories, Tributes, and Perspectives

Former students of Carol B. Pratt fondly remember his idiosyncrasies and remarkable intellect, as well as his inventive and unique, yet practical, approaches to optometric science and clinical care. The following anecdotes and remembrances illustrate his strong mathematical bent, mischievous sense of humor, occasional eccentricities, positive impact on his students, and the respect students and colleagues had for him.

"IN THROUGH THERE"

Many lecturers have a phrase that they repeat frequently, most likely unconsciously. Pratt often used the phrase "in through there," particularly while pointing to an illustration, a graph, or numerical data. For example, several of his uses of this phrase were found in a lecture that was recorded on DVD. When he was talking about a graph of myopia as a function of age, for a patient in which the rates of myopia progression were different in the two eyes, he observed that: "We have an increased anisometropia in through there." When he presented another graph that involved a patient who had typical childhood myopia progression, with stabilization in the teens, he said that: "The myopia stabilized at about 3.25 diopters in through there."[1] In another lecture when he was talking about astigmatism, he pointed out that: "I shifted the axis ten degrees in through there."[2]

PRATT'S JEFFERSON HALL OFFICE

Visitors to Pratt's office in Jefferson Hall, home of the College of Optometry, were typically struck by the jumbled piles of books and papers on his desk; the chalkboard filled with numbers, formulas, and notes written at all angles to fit in the available space; and, at the back of his large office, an examination chair, stand with Bausch & Lomb Greens' Refractor, and Bausch & Lomb projector.

Members of the College of Optometry Class of 1970 recall an incident involving Pratt's chalkboard. The tangle of numbers and formulas was obviously part of some ongoing calculations, as the word SAVE was written in the upper left-hand corner of the chalkboard. At the beginning of one early morning lecture class, Pratt came into the classroom muttering and appearing a little upset. When asked about it, he revealed that the new janitor had erased the entire chalkboard, except for the word SAVE.

PRATT'S "INTERESTING RELATIONSHIP WITH MATHEMATICS"

Pratt's youngest son, Jeff, observed that his father "had an interesting relationship with mathematics."[3] Ted Dorn, a member of the College of Optometry Class of 1970, remembered Pratt working physiological optics problems on the chalkboard, and coming up with answers "with fractions like 13/57. Then he would divide it out in his head to about three decimal places, then say 'somewhere in through there' (with a snicker). I figured he had it all memorized because that would be too difficult to do in your head."[4] Considering how comfortable Pratt was with mathematics, one has to wonder whether he did do that in his head.

It may be noted that optics and mathematics were important in the vocations of other Pratt family members. As discussed in chapter 1, Pratt's father, George, was an optometrist. Pratt's younger sister, Norabel Pratt

Miller, was a math instructor at Pacific University.[5] His youngest son, Jeff, worked for over 40 years in ophthalmic lens laboratory management software.[3]

One manifestation of Pratt's relationship with mathematics was his fondness for detailed graphs. Former students of Pratt can readily recall him drawing graphs on the chalkboard or presenting graphs on transparencies using an overhead projector. Appendix 3 presents two graphs drawn by Pratt, illustrating how he liked to produce graphs packed with data.

THE GRADING SYSTEM

Pratt's son, Jeff, remembers a story that his father told about students who were overly concerned about grades, and who asked him repeatedly how he determined grades. Pratt didn't care much about grades; he was more interested in having students learn. He answered that he took all the exam papers in one hand, and, standing at the top of the stairs, he threw them all down the stairwell. Those that went all the way down got Cs, those that went halfway down got Bs, and the ones that stayed near the top got As.

PRATT STORIES FROM WILLARD BLEYTHING

Willard Bleything earned three degrees from Pacific University, his undergraduate degree, his O.D. degree in 1952, and an M.S. in 1954. Bleything has had a distinguished career in optometry, including sixteen years in private practice, serving as president of the Oregon optometry board, and a long stint as Dean of the College of Optometry. Bleything attended Pacific University before Jefferson Hall was built for optometry. He recalled having an optics class with Pratt in the basement of McCormick

Hall. It was a long narrow classroom with a low riser for the professor to stand on. Pratt paced the width of the riser continually, always deep in thoughts and calculations. Everyone expected Pratt to misstep one day and fall off the edge, but he never did.[6]

Bleything also remembered serving as a teaching assistant for Pratt and helping him with some of his novel experiments on vision. One memorable experiment involved trying to find out if spinning affected convergence. Pratt had a chair and stand rigged up on a circular platform that could be rotated 360 degrees. Bleything and other teaching assistants walked around in a circle rotating the platform while Pratt did testing on subjects seated in the chair on the platform. The experiment did not yield a meaningful result, and Bleything recalls that the assistants got tired and a little dizzy.

PRATT'S AVANTI

Pacific University students from the 1960s remember Pratt's Studebaker Avanti automobile. Studebaker made the Avanti in 1962 and 1963. It had a very distinctive and futuristic style. Pratt loved his Avanti for its look, but possibly also for its supercharged engine because he accumulated more than one speeding ticket during his long commutes to Forest Grove from his home.[6]

A STORY FROM PRATT

In 1970, the Oregon Optometrist published some recollections of the early days of the optometry school at Pacific University as a celebration of its 25th anniversary.[7] Pratt offered the following anecdote:

"I remember when our first sizable class was about ready for clinical experience. I phoned the business manager, Mr. Shumm, and told him we couldn't continue with only two refractors for use – we needed an additional fourteen of them. When he asked what they cost I told him seven-fifty and he said that was OK, if that was all, to purchase them. I forgot to mention that the seven-fifty was $750 each – we got the phoropters and there was a large hemorrhage in the office upstairs for a while, since this was double our annual budget."[8]

REMEMBRANCES FROM BOB EDWARDS

Bob Edwards was a 1971 graduate of Pacific University College of Optometry. He called Pratt "the most brilliant professor I ever had."[9] Edwards recalled that he started having headaches and a great deal of difficulty reading in his second year in optometry school. A student clinician examined him in clinic but was uncertain in his analysis of the test findings. The student clinician arranged for Edwards to be examined by Pratt in his office. Edwards recalled that Pratt "did the most amazing exam I have ever had. Nearly all of the visual findings were taken at near and extrapolated to distance. This was not a visual acuity exam. This was different."[9] Pratt went over the graph of the test results with the student clinician and Edwards, and prescribed: OD, +0.25 D sphere, with ¾ prism diopter base-out; OS, +0.50 -0.25 x 180, with ¾ prism diopter base-out; and +0.75 D add for near. With that prescription, Edwards said that: "My headaches were over. I could study again....This experience with Dr. Pratt shaped my whole career."[9] In particular, Edwards credited Pratt with giving him confidence in prescribing prism and inspiring his work in neuro-optometric rehabilitation.

Edwards also related experiences with Pratt's lectures. He said that students became accustomed to Pratt's "chicken scratch writing, goatee stroking, and cackling laugh." One physiological optics lecture was particularly memorable. Pratt started writing on the upper left-hand corner of the left-most of three chalkboards at the front of the room. He proceeded to fill all three boards with calculations and then moved to the chalkboard on the right-hand wall of the classroom. Pratt finally completed the calculations in the lower right corner of that last remaining chalkboard, having used all four blackboards to derive a simplified ocular optics formula and constants. Edwards said that Pratt challenged his physics and math backgrounds, but Edwards "is grateful for the knowledge he imparted to me and the curiosity he instilled."[9]

Another story told by Bob Edwards illustrates Pratt's good nature and patience toward students. Edwards worked with his classmate Rod Helm on their fourth-year research project, with Pratt as their advisor. Pratt suggested an experiment with vertical stenopaic slits. After carefully testing a large number of subjects, analyzing the data, and writing up the results, they met with Pratt to discuss the outcome of their study. Pratt was perplexed that their results differed so much from what he expected, even though the data were fairly consistent. Pratt asked them to explain again how they did the experiment. When Pratt realized that they put the stenopaic slits in front of both eyes, "he reared back in his chair, tipped his head, and released a huge cackling laugh. This was followed by a right knee slap and an uncontrolled session of laughter and knee-slapping. 'You were supposed to put the slit in front of one eye.'"[9] Pratt did not chastise them for their mistake and accepted their work as completing the course requirement, apparently recognizing their good faith efforts on the experiment.

THE "MERRY CHRISTMAS" MULTIPLE CHOICE EXAM

Pratt was known for the difficult examinations he gave. The examination Pratt gave in December, 1969 in his physiological optics class is prominent in Pratt lore among his former students. The fact that he rarely gave multiple choice tests is only part of the story. First person accounts from Bob Edwards and other members of his class differed slightly on some of the details of the test, but their input made it possible to assemble a narrative of that event.[9,10]

The two-hour test was given in December just before Christmas break. There were less than twenty problems, each with multiple choice answers. As usual with a Pratt test, they were difficult problems requiring many calculations. The possible answers for the first questions were labeled q, r, s, and t. At the time, Edwards speculated that must have been a mistake, but after extensive calculation, he selected s, and went ahead to the next question. Possible answers for the second question were a, b, c, and d. Answers to choose from on the third question were m, n, o, and p.

Meanwhile, Pratt was drawing a holly leaf and berries on the chalkboard, then writing Merry Christmas 1969, and then drawing another holly leaf and berries. Edwards was among the last few students to leave the room after the exam. One of the students told Pratt that it was a difficult exam, and wanted to know when the answers would be available. Pratt answered that he had put the answers on the chalkboard an hour ago. The answer key was Merry Christmas spelled backwards!

This test was given in the days before scantron answer sheets, and students wrote their answers to the left of each question. One could imagine an astute student seeing the pattern emerging on the page. The next semester, in class, Pratt acknowledged the student who got the best score on the test, by missing only one question on the test. One could conclude that with no perfect scores on the test, no one cracked the code of the key.

ADMIRATION FROM FORMER STUDENTS

John Rush, a 1969 optometry graduate, remembers Pratt's phrase "in through there," and said that: "To this day, I find myself repeating that phrase at the end of a point I'm making. I'm not sure why except that maybe to remind myself of what a good prof he was and how he impacted many of us."[11]

Don James, Class of 1970, who was a lab instructor for Pratt in his fourth year of optometry school said that: "I really enjoyed and admired him and can still picture the 'sparkle in his eye' when he smiled."[12] James also remembered that Pratt's car was usually quite dirty, and that one day he and some classmates surprised Pratt by washing it.

PERSPECTIVE FROM A PRATT PATIENT

Even though Pratt retired more than 45 years ago, it was possible to contact a former patient through Pratt's son Jeff. Patty took the bus to work on her lengthy daily commute from her home east of Portland into downtown Portland. Jeff was one of her fellow riders on his way to downtown Portland.

As they got to know each other, Jeff noticed that Patty had some eye problems. She had worn glasses since she was six years old, but none of her prescriptions, over the years, had been totally satisfying. She thought that was just the way it was going to be.

Jeff invited her to meet his dad, who he thought might be able to help her. He knew his dad's eye exams were very thorough and that he used a different approach than most of the other doctors used. Dr. Pratt was retired by this time in the mid-1970s, but he had a full exam set up, with exam chair, stand, and an old B&L Greens' refractor, at their house. Even though he was retired, he still liked to play around with testing strategies.

Eventually, Patty made it to the Pratt house, at first for a social visit, and then, later for an eye exam. Patty said they developed a "very kindly relationship." At first, Patty didn't know quite how to address Dr. Pratt. Jeff said, "Just call him Doc. That's what everyone at the bar calls him."

After the exam, Dr. Pratt suggested a glasses frame, from a small inventory he had, and he had some glasses made for her. She said that it was "the best correction she'd had" since needing glasses twenty years before.

Patty said that "Doc" did many more tests than the other doctors she had seen previously. She observed that it was as though he didn't just want to come up with a pair of glasses for her, but that he wanted to understand as much as possible how her vision worked. That, of course, was the basis for the Pratt examination procedure – to understand the patient's visual system, knowing that every visual system is unique.

TRIBUTES FROM PACIFIC UNIVERSITY FACULTY COLLEAGUES

Evidence for the respect and appreciation that faculty at Pacific University, both in Optometry and other departments, had for Pratt can be found in the November-December, 1966 issue of the Oregon Optometrist.[13] Harold Haynes, a long-time optometry faculty member at Pacific University, said: "His concepts of professional rather than technical education for optometrists have materially shaped the evolution of the faculty's thinking and our curriculum. He is foremost in our group discussions in articulating the blending of the humanism of the liberal arts tradition, the contribution of the basic sciences, and the unique necessities of the clinical in the development of our academic program. He has been singularly instrumental in helping to develop the best thinking from his colleagues by shrewd debate and kindly suggestions. I often feel that all too few outside the university community realize the modesty, patience, and brilliance of this scholar."

John Roberts, Pacific University Professor of Biology observed that: "Hundreds of students have passed through his classes. Each student has probably 'griped' due to the exactness which he expects in a classroom situation, however these same students when they get out in practice throw bouquets at Carol and are glad that they've had the experience of working with this outstanding teacher. This high regard as a teacher draws respect and admiration from all those on the faculty."[13]

J. Russell Roberts, Professor of English at Pacific University, stated that: "Each of us in his own way finds his place in the University scene as a teacher, counselor, and scholar. Carol in his way as a teacher, counselor, and scholar has shaped the University personnel program, the curriculum, and the liaison between faculty and administration; but above all, by being present, always in a quiet way, he lends a kind of presence to any gathering that promises a thoughtful, witty, conciliatory solution of fretful issues."[13]

PERSONAL NOTE FROM SCOTT PIKE

Dr. Pratt's lectures could be very technical, with lots of math and graphs. His speaking volume would rise and fall, sometimes dropping into a mumble when he was doing math on the fly, in his head. This pattern of speech required one to pay close attention at all times. Those technical lectures were very challenging for me. But, in our final semester with Dr. Pratt, when he presented cases from his practice, my attention to his words was tuned to high.

I was especially struck by his presentation of the two patients who had decreases in myopia associated with radical alterations in their lives (discussed in Chapter 5). Dr. Pratt went into fairly deep detail describing the visual patterns and case histories for both of these patients. He brought these two stories together in the end by illustrating the similarities both patients showed in their visual patterns before and after their life-changing choices. With data, graphs, and case history details, Dr. Pratt showed us that stress from different sources can have a dramatic influence on the visual system.

For me, after this lecture, patients were no longer just a couple of eyeballs behind a phoropter. I had to consider the whole of the patient to really understand the stresses on his or her visual system. Dr. Pratt's lecture flashed in my mind at times, in practice, when I would encounter grade school children with accommodative problems, and also living through a divorce at home. Or, when I was working with keratoconus patients at times when their corneas were changing, I might inquire what else was going on in their lives. Often there were financial problems, marriage problems, legal problems, or other stress-inducing situations.

While Dr. Pratt was a genius at crunching the data gathered from an in-depth eye exam, he also had great wisdom to see patients from a broader perspective, at the human level with all of life's twists and turns, bumps and jolts. One of the things about Dr. Pratt's methods that stuck with me through the years was his ability to take all his results, treat them in his own special and sometimes complex ways and still be very practical in deriving an Rx. His greater gift may have been to present all this to his students in a meaningful way so that his insights would travel to people in towns and cities beyond his immediate reach.

PERSONAL NOTE FROM DAVID GOSS

My years as a student at Pacific University coincided with Pratt's last years as a faculty member before his retirement. My class did not have a lecture course from Pratt. At that time, he was one of the supervising optometrists at the College of Optometry's Portland clinic, and he had an aniseikonia special clinic at the Forest Grove clinic. I was one of a handful of students who frequented his office to observe him testing patients or demonstrating testing techniques, and I took an elective course with him on case analysis. I also watched many of the videotapes of lectures he gave in 1971, taking copious notes, and even recording some of them on audiotapes for later review. My fascination with his study on myopia progression spurred me to make myopia the primary focus of my research for the first twenty years of my career.

I admired many of our other optometry school instructors, but Pratt truly stood out. One reason was that he seemed to have information that could not be obtained elsewhere. Perhaps a bigger reason for me was that while our other instructors were primarily, or entirely, either clinicians or researchers, Pratt was both. The synergy of his integration of clinical practice and research was appealing and seemed to be an ideal way to be able to incorporate research into day-to-day patient care. He used test findings from routine examinations of his patients as research data to inform the design of his examination procedures and to describe the natural history of clinical conditions, leading ultimately to better patient care.

REMEMBRANCE OF PRATT FROM HAROLD HAYNES

Harold Haynes gave a touching eulogy for Pratt.[14] In 1948, Haynes was the third full-time optometry faculty member hired at Pacific (Pratt was the first in 1945 and Detleff Jans the second in 1947). At the time of his hiring, Haynes was 23 years old, 17 years younger than Pratt. Pratt sensed that Haynes, as an insecure young faculty member, had some concern about the possibility of the two of them having some differences in their theoretical and clinical viewpoints. Pratt proposed that they take ten cases and compare their analyses. Haynes found this to be "a humane and scholarly way to relieve my anxiety – a perfect way to establish a professional relationship." They went on to have a strong friendship, with them often discussing optometric education at Pratt's acreage.

Haynes characterized Pratt as "a kind and compassionate man," who "always found the time to help a colleague, a troubled student, a patient, a staff member, or friend."[14] Haynes recalled an occasion when he asked Pratt why he left biophysics research for optometry and why he chose to teach optometry. Pratt answered that he wanted to help people rather than spending the rest of his life in the laboratory, and that by training students, he could help more people than he could solely in private practice. For these reasons and more, Haynes said that colleagues and students sometimes called Pratt Mr. Optometry.[14]

A CONTINUING LEGACY

Pratt retired from teaching roughly a half-century ago, and it is concerning that he seems to be forgotten. However, one can find occasional glimpses of his influence even from optometrists who were not among his students. Michelle Monkman, a 1992 graduate of the Pacific University College of Optometry and former president of the Oregon Board of Optometry, practices in Pendleton, Oregon. When she was a student, Richard Septon, a devotee of Pratt testing and analysis procedures, taught the case analysis course. Septon spent time in class on Pratt graphing methods and the importance of binocular vision tests. Monkman also had Septon as an attending doctor in clinic. Septon required his clinic students to graph their results. Monkman said that the graphing gave her added confidence in her prescriptions, rather than just looking at 7A and paying little attention to other findings, as some staff doctors did.[15] That lesson gave her a better basis for her examinations in practice.[15] She also makes regular use of the Pratt nearpoint card.[15] It is stories such as Monkman's that show that Pratt's positive impact does extend beyond his immediate students.

References

1. Pratt CB. Videotaped lecture, March 8, 1971, Pacific University videotape VT50 (also recorded on DVD).
2. Pratt CB. Videotaped lecture, September 10, 1971, Pacific University videotape VT68.
3. Pratt J. Telephone call with Scott Pike, October 12, 2020.
4. Dorn T. Email to Scott Pike, January, 2021.
5. Pratt J. Email to Scott Pike, November, 2020.
6. Bleything W. Interview by Scott Pike, November, 2020.
7. Baker WJ, ed. The twenty-fifth anniversary of the College of Optometry at Pacific University. Oregon Optometrist 1970;37(6):4-25.
8. Pratt CB. And the pains of progress were tinged with humor. Oregon Optometrist 1970;37(6):8.
9. Edwards B. Email to Scott Pike, February, 2021.

10. Weisenbach J. Email to Scott Pike, May, 2021.
11. Rush J. Email to Scott Pike, February, 2021.
12. James D. Email to Scott Pike, February, 2021.
13. Roberts J, Roberts JR, Haynes HM. As they see Carol Pratt. Oregon Optometrist. Nov.-Dec., 1966:5-6.
14. Haynes HM. In Memory of a Friend. Handwritten copy of a eulogy read at memorial services at Oregon City, Oregon, March 16, 1984.
15. Monkman M. Telephone call with Scott Pike, May, 2021.

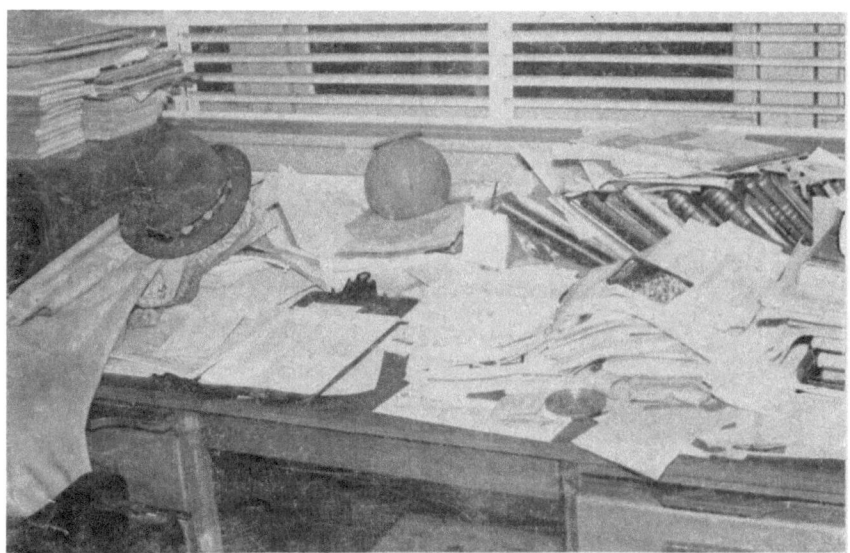

Figure 6.1. A photograph of Pratt's desk in his office in Jefferson Hall on the Pacific University campus, taken from the front cover of the November-December, 1966 issue of The Oregon Optometrist. (Image courtesy Oregon Optometric Physicians Association)

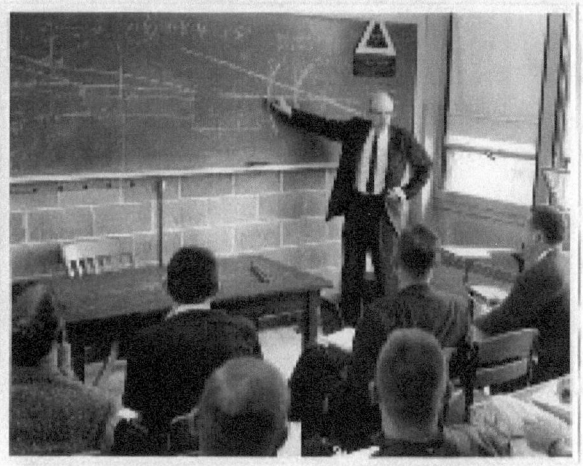

Figure 6.2. Carol Pratt giving a lecture in the College of Optometry's Jefferson Hall. It appears that he is solving an optics problem. (Image courtesy Pacific University Archives)

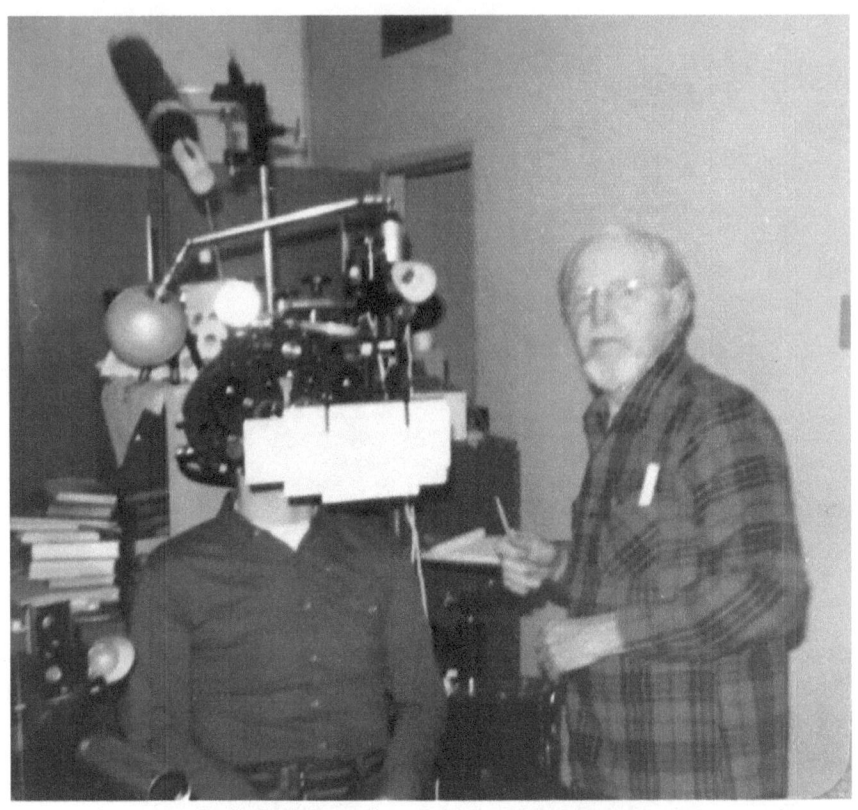

Figure 6.3. Pratt demonstrating testing procedures in his third floor Jefferson Hall office with a student as patient, December, 1974. (Photo from David Goss)

Appendix 1

List of Tests in the OEP 21-point Examination

In the 1920s and 1930s, A. M. Skeffington and associates developed a examination sequence of 21 tests.[1,2,3] It built on Charles Sheard's 1917 list of 18 tests to be done in an optometric examination.[4,5,6] Skeffington was Director of Education for the Optometric Extension Program (OEP) and most of his writings were published by OEP. The 21 test sequence came to be known as the OEP 21-point examination. It was used by many optometrists when Pratt went into practice in 1936 and for many years thereafter. The following table lists the tests in that examination procedure. Pratt used this routine for only about his first six months of practice, but throughout his subsequent career he usually referred to various tests by their OEP test numbers.

Skeffington and associates also developed a system for analyzing the accommodation and convergence test findings in the 21-point exam. That analysis procedure came to be known as OEP analysis.[2,3,7,8] Other analysis systems were developed using graphical procedures, comparisons to norms, and various rules of thumb.[9] Pratt designed his own unique examination sequence, described in Chapter 2 and Appendix 2, and his own unique method of analyzing accommodation and convergence findings, described in Chapter 3.

Test number	Test description
1	Ophthalmoscopy
2	Ophthalmometry (keratometry)

3	Habitual lateral dissociated phoria at distance
13A	Habitual lateral dissociated phoria at near
4	Static retinoscopy
5	Dynamic retinoscopy at 20 inches (50 cm)
6	Dynamic retinoscopy at 40 inches (1 m)
7	Subjective refraction: maximum plus to 20/20 minus visual acuity
7A	Subjective refraction: maximum plus to best visual acuity
8	Lateral dissociated phoria at distance through #7 finding
9	Base-out to first blur fusional vergence range at distance
10	Base-out to break and recovery fusional vergence range at distance
11	Base-in to break and recovery fusional vergence range at distance
12	Vertical dissociated phoria and fusional vergence ranges at distance
13B	Lateral dissociated phoria at near through #7 finding
14A	Unfused (monocular) cross cylinder
15A	Lateral dissociated phoria at near through the #14A finding
14B	Fused (binocular) cross cylinder
15B	Lateral dissociated phoria at near through the #14B finding

16A	Base-out to blur out fusional vergence range at near
16B	Base-out to break and recovery fusional vergence range at near
17A	Base-in to blur out fusional vergence range at near
17B	Base-in to break and recovery fusional vergence range at near
18	Vertical dissociated phoria and fusional vergence ranges at near
19	Analytical amplitude (minus to blur with card at 13 inches)
20	Binocular minus-to-blur-out with card at 16 inches
21	Binocular plus-to-blur-out with card at 16 inches

References

1. Skeffington AM. Differential Diagnosis in Ocular Examination. Chicago: A. J. Cox, 1931.
2. Lesser SK. Fundamentals of Procedure and Analysis, 3rd ed. Fort Worth, TX: S. K. Lesser, 1933.
3. Birnbaum MH. Optometric Management of Nearpoint Vision Disorders. Boston: Butterworth-Heinemann, 1993:121-160.
4. Sheard C. Dynamic Ocular Tests. Columbus, OH: Lawrence Press, 1917.
5. Borish IM. 21 points. Newsletter Optom Hist Soc 1987;18:23-24.
6. Hendrickson H. 21 points and more. Newsletter Optom Hist Soc 1987;18:55-56.
7. Pheiffer CH. Analytical Analysis of A. M. Skeffington, O.D. and Associates. Duncan, OK: Optometric Extension Program, 1981.
8. Schmitt EP. Guidelines for Clinical Testing, Lens Prescribing, and Vision Care. Santa Ana, CA: Optometric Extension Program, 1996.
9. Borish IM. Clinical Refraction, 3rd ed. Chicago, IL: Professional Press, 1970:861-937.

Appendix 2

Pratt's Examination Sequence

The testing sequence which Pratt used for most of his years in practice, starting in the early 1940s, is as follows:

1) The first test performed was keratometry. Testing with the phoropter was done after keratometry.

    The "behind the phoropter" tests begin with testing at near (16" or 40 cm.) using full nearpoint illumination and a nearpoint card. The phoropter Pratt used was a Bausch & Lomb Greens' Refractor.

2) Start with the patient being able to read 20/30 or better on the nearpoint card. With the case history, visual acuity findings, keratometry results, and/or previous patient findings, this starting point can easily be found. Add plus monocularly to blur out and recovery (21m test). Repeat binocularly. (NRA)

3) Next is the Pratt near cylinder test for astigmatism, done monocularly. Using the previous recovery and assuming the astigmatic axes for most patients are close to vertical or horizontal (check keratometer reading), start with the horizontal/vertical cross grid card. Ask the patient which lines appear blacker and more distinct, "up and down or across." Set the axis in the phoropter 90 degrees from the lines reported blacker. Add cylinder power, maintaining sphere equivalent, until the patient reports the lines are equal in blackness or the blackness reverses.

    Next, present the oblique cross grid card and ask which lines are blacker and more distinct. Turn the axis dial, using a bracketing method, until the lines are equal in blackness. This will be done by turning the dial "away" from the orientation of the blacker lines until equal.

Return to the horizontal/vertical cross grid card and double check for equal blackness. Re-adjust, if necessary. Then repeat for the other eye.

4) Using the results of the previous test, perform unfused cross cylinder tests on each eye and do a phoria test through the endpoint. (OEP 14A and 15A)

5) With rotary prisms in place test the base-in vergence ranges (blur, break and recovery). (OEP 17A and 17B) At the breakpoint ask if the targets are level (indication of vertical deviation).

Return the prism setting in the phoropter to 16 Δ BI. Even if the recovery value is low, adding a click or two of plus should allow the patient to clear 20/20. Check for singleness of vision.

6) Add plus lenses binocularly to blur out and recovery. Recovery is reached when the patient can read 2/3 of the 20/20 line. (OEP 21 with 16 Δ BI)

7) With 16 Δ BI still in place, put the phoropter cross cylinder lenses, oriented obliquely, into position for testing and show the patient the oblique cross grid target. Perform a fused crossed cylinder test, stopping at equality or reversal if no equal response. (OEP 14B with 16 Δ BI)

8) Remove the base-in prism and repeat a cross cylinder test. The starting lenses are the endpoint lenses from the previous test. (OEP 14B)

9) Put the prisms back in place and measure the base-out vergence ranges, recording blur, break and recovery. Ask the patient to report any change in apparent size or distance (SILO effect). (OEP 16A and 16B)

Add prism base-out to a total of 10 Δ BO and check acuity.

10) With 10 Δ base-out in place put the cross cylinder lenses in place, set obliquely, and do another fused cross cylinder test. (OEP 14B with 10 Δ BO)

Pratt's Examination Sequence

11) Remove the cross cylinder lenses and add more base-out prism and/or more minus lenses power to cause increased accommodative and convergence stimulation. The amount of stimulation depends on how much the patient can handle. Have the patient clear the bottom line to provide a longer period of stimulation.

12) Reposition the cross cylinder lenses, and return the prisms to 10 Δ BO. Now, repeat a cross cylinder test approaching equality from the minus side. (-14B with 10 Δ BO)

13) Immediately rotate the prisms back to zero and remove them. With the cross cylinder lenses still in place, repeat the cross cylinder test measuring from the minus side. (-14B)

Note: Steps 10 through 13 are not done on presbyopes, as all cross cylinder test values will be close to the same due to reduced accommodation abilities.

14) Add minus lenses to blur out and recovery. (PRA or OEP 20)

Note: Later in his career, Pratt did not drive accommodation to blur out in 0.25 D steps, but rather he clicked in -4.00 D at this point using the 4 D step master lens disc in the Greens' Refractor. And then he reduced minus in 0.25 D steps to the recovery.

At this point an estimation of the distance refraction can be made by averaging the values for NRA with 16 Δ BI minus 3.25 and 14B with 16 Δ BI minus 2.00. (From step 6 and step 7 above). This average is referred to as P_2, which is equal to:

$$\frac{(\text{NRA with } 16\ \Delta\ \text{BI} - 3.25) + (14\text{B with } 16\ \Delta\ \text{BI} - 2.00)}{2}$$

Next, Dr. Pratt did two series of phorias and vergences, using P_2 as the base for the control lens.

15) Using the control lens of $P_2 - 0.50$ D:
   a. Do a standard near phoria
   b. Do a BI vergence range (OEP 17A, 17B). At the recovery point,

have the patient read the bottom line, reducing the BI value, if necessary, for clarity.

c. Immediately repeat a standard near phoria.

Using the control lens of $P_2 + 0.50$ D:

d. Do a standard near phoria

e. Do a BO vergence range (OEP 16A, 16B). At the recovery point, have the patient read the bottom line, reducing the BO value, if necessary, for clarity.

f. Immediately repeat a standard near phoria.

16) Move the target distance to approximately 28 cm. (11") and add plus, if necessary, to be sure the next cross cylinder test is begun from the plus side. Have the patient read the letters before beginning the test. Then add the obliquely oriented cross-cylinder lenses and perform another binocular cross cylinder (14B), followed by a phoria at the same distance.

17) Move the nearpoint target back to 40 cm. and do a standard cross cylinder test.

THIS CONCLUDES THE SEQUENCE OF NEAR TESTS.

18) Bichrome test: Setting the phoropter for distance testing, display the bichrome (red-green) target using the 20/40 size letters. Using P_2 as a control lens, start by adding 0.50 D of plus power so that the bichrome is started from the plus side. Do the test OD, OS, OU, recording the equal point, or if there is no equal, the eighth diopter between the lens powers before and after reversal.

19) Far cross cylinder: Replace the bichrome target with sets of oblique lines (the oblique T on the Bausch & Lomb projector). Add 0.25 D to the phoropter and with the cross cylinder lenses in place (oriented

obliquely), do a cross cylinder test at far. Record the equal point, or if there is no equal, the eighth diopter between the lens powers before and after reversal.

20) Blur in at far: Remove the cross cylinder lenses and display the 20/40 letters on the distance chart. These letters should be very clear. Add plus to just short of a total blur out. Next, display the 20/20 letters, which will be blurred. Instruct the patient that you are going to change the lenses. Instruct the patient to report when he/she can first read most of the 20/20 letters. The letters don't have to be sharp and clear, just when he/she can make out most of them. Record this binocular finding.

The next step is to calculate the final P-factor, which is equal to:

$$\frac{(21 \text{ w}/16\text{BI} - 3.25) + (14\text{B w}/16\text{BI} - 2.00) + \text{Bichrome} + (\text{Far CC} + 0.25) + (\text{Blur-in} - 0.50)}{5}$$

21) If P falls in between quarter diopter steps in the phoropter, check the lenses on either side of P, for the best subjective response for clarity. Check the visual acuities and record the final refraction.
22) Do a standard far phoria
23) Do a standard base in vergence range at far.
24) Do a standard base out vergence range at far.

That concludes the examination. Some of the important qualities of this examination procedure, including logic, ease of flow, and fullness of the exam, are the following:

1) The comprehensive nature of the exam is shown by the number of tests that deal not just with a distance refraction, but also with the interrelationships of accommodation and convergence. In Dr. Pratt's view, this is where the complexities of the visual system lie – where

important visual problems are found. An optometrist experienced with a retinoscope can arrive at a distance refraction quickly, but that says nothing about the workings of the accommodation and convergence systems. If a distance refraction is your only goal or endpoint, then you may be missing important information. Many vision problems stem from inefficiencies in accommodation and/or convergence.

2) The examination is very dynamic. The stimulation and inhibition of the accommodation and convergence systems during the exam reproduce the demands on the visual system that individuals may face in their daily life. The fullness of the exam helps to show how the visual system reacts to different presets, and how an individual reacts to fatigue, as may occur from doing close work all day long.

3) The flow of the exam is continuous going from an inhibited state (plus and base in) to a stimulated state (minus and base out). One test easily flows into the next.

4) Having a prediction of the distance refraction before distance testing begins is also an advantage to the flow of the exam because testing often bogs down in distance testing when it is done first.

5) Another advantage of this testing procedure is that the exam contains fewer "blurry choices" which are difficult for many patients to make.

6) With the P-factor information, we have a refraction estimation based on five approximations, rather than one or two. This averaging makes the estimation of the refraction more accurate.

7) Pratt did this exam sequence thousands of times in the 1940's, 50's and 60's when patients generally didn't live at the frenetic pace that so many people live today, and they seemingly valued completeness and quality more than people today when quickness and convenience seem to have a very high priority. Long exam times were not uncommon. Today it is difficult to have a patient sit still long enough for all these tests, and as insurance payments sometimes dictate, a doctor may not be able to afford the time required for an extended exam as

Pratt did.

However, one can trim the exam to a shorter form, which still includes basic accommodative and convergence findings. One can omit steps 10 through 13 and steps 15 through 17 listed above. On average patients with prompt responses, time behind the phoropter with this shortened exam is usually under 10 minutes. The more extreme stimulations and inhibitions to the visual system included in the full exam can be saved for patients with greater visual system difficulties.

Appendix 3

Accommodation and Convergence Graphs Plotted by Pratt

Although Pratt must have plotted thousands of accommodation and convergence graphs, very few examples of ones he plotted himself survive. Two such examples are provided here for the purpose of illustrating Pratt's fondness for complicated graphs jammed with information.

Figure A3.1 is a screen-shot from a DVD which had been transferred from a videotape of one of Pratt's lectures at Pacific University, probably in 1971. The exact date of the lecture is unknown. The quality of the image is poor, but its clarity may be similar to that experienced by students in the back row of the classroom after the chalk had been smeared by the back of Pratt's hand and the points re-plotted a time or two. Figure A3.1 is a graph of the means from many different studies over several years in his practice. Testing procedures, test distances, illumination levels, prism settings for cross cylinder tests, lens pre-sets for cross cylinder tests, and lens powers for dissociated phorias were varied in the different studies. Such a graph may have been one of Pratt's steps in deriving his normative data.

Pratt plotted the graph in Figure A3.1 in chalk on a blackboard that had a grid for drawing graphs. The authors have added labels to the graph. The horizontal line with A just beneath it is the x-axis on which accommodation in diopters is plotted. The vertical line with C just to its left is the y-axis on which convergence in meter angles is plotted. PH is at the top of the phoria line on which separate mean phoria points are plotted with Xs. CC is at the top of the cross cylinder line on which separate mean cross cylinder points are plotted with circles, squares, and diamonds. NRA is just to the left of the band going through plus-to-blur-out (negative relative accommodation) points. PRA is just to the right of the band going through minus-to-blur-out (positive relative accommodation) points. The horizontal line segments at various places on the graph are likely base-in and base-out break and recovery fusional vergence findings.

Figure A3.2 is a graph Pratt plotted in 1957. He did not label anything on the graph, but his usual method of plotting accommodation and convergence can be discerned, points marked with Xs being phorias and points marked with open circles being cross cylinders. The three cross cylinders plotted side by side at one convergence level likely represent cross cylinders with plus and minus pre-sets and another repeated later in the exam. It also appears that he plotted fusional vergence ranges and relative accommodation findings in Figure 3.2, which have been labeled based on the authors' interpretations.

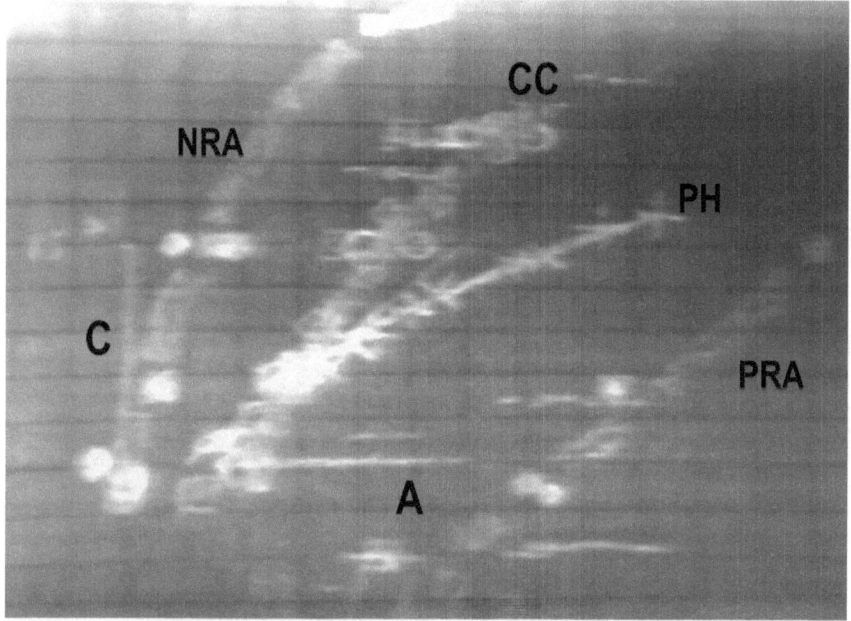

Figure A3.1. Graph plotted by Pratt in one of his lectures at Pacific University with points representing means from many statistical studies he did based on patient data from his practice. From study to study Pratt varied testing procedures, test distances, illumination levels, prism settings, and lens settings. Labels added based on interpretation of the graph by the authors: A, x-axis, accommodation in diopters; C, y-axis, convergence in meter angles; PH, phoria line; CC, cross cylinder line; NRA, negative relative accommodation; PRA, positive relative accommodation. The quality of this image is poor, but it does provide an illustration of Pratt's predilection for highly detailed graphs with numerous data points. Bright spots on the graph resulted from several overlapping data points, the brightest spot apparently at the intersection of phoria and cross cylinder lines. (Image from a screen-shot by the authors from a DVD of a Pratt lecture, date unknown, probably 1971)

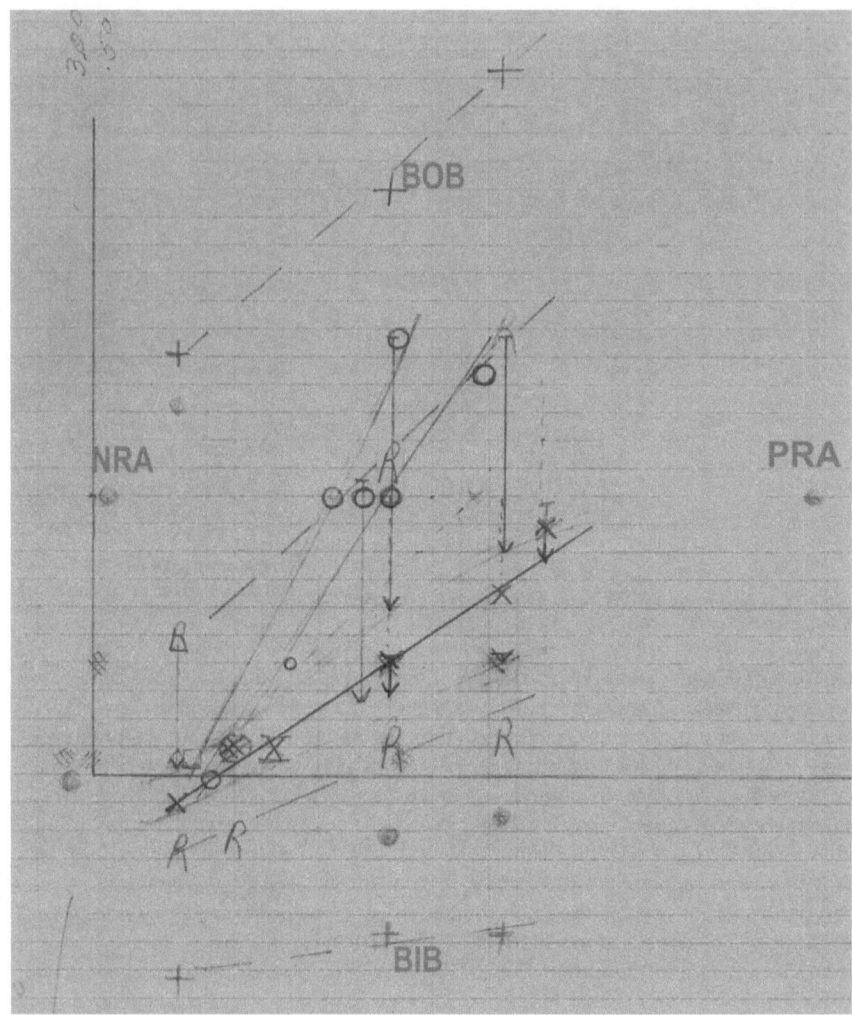

Figure A3.2. Accommodation (x-axis) and convergence (y-axis) graph plotted on paper by Pratt in 1957. Points marked with Xs are phorias and points marked with open circles are cross cylinders. Filled circles are NRA and PRA points. Plus signs are fusional vergence break points. Points marked with Rs are likely recovery points on fusional vergence range testing. Labels based on the authors' interpretation of the graph: BIB, base-in break; BOB, base-out break; NRA, negative relative accommodation; PRA, positive relative accommodation. (Image of a document provided by Jeffrey Pratt)

Appendix 4

Pratt Accommodation and Convergence Norms

Patrick Davidson and William Meyer, in their O.D. thesis, gave numerical values for Pratt norms for binocular cross cylinder, negative relative accommodation, and positive relative accommodation at four convergence stimulus levels, and for phoria, base-in break and recovery, and base-out break and recovery at four accommodative stimulus levels.[1] No explanation was given in the Davidson and Meyer thesis concerning derivation of the norms. The values are plotted in Figure A4.1. It may be noted that the placement of the points on the graph is very similar to that of the mean data from the Pike study plotted in Figure 3.6.

References

1. Davidson PS, Meyer WR. An interpretation of Pratt analytical techniques and comparison of near-point therapy to that of O. E. P. O.D. thesis, Pacific University, 1973.

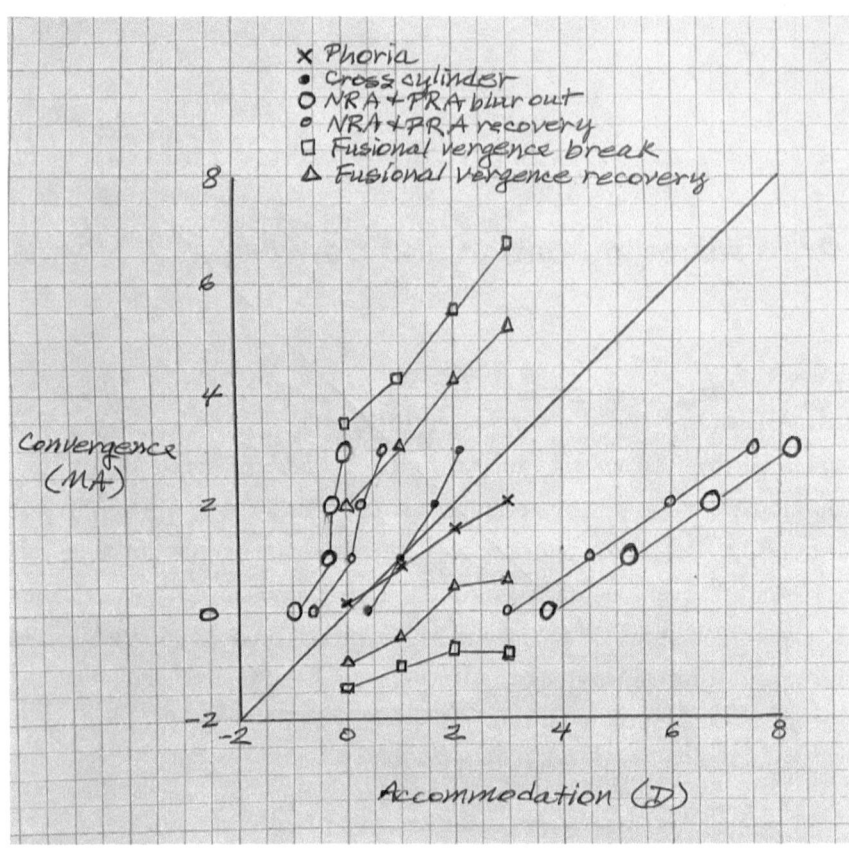

Figure A4.1. Graph of Pratt norms given in the Davidson and Meyer O.D. thesis. Plotted values were adjusted for vertex distance. (Graph plotted by the authors)

Appendix 5

Pratt's Method of Aniseikonia Measurement

Pratt devised a method for measuring aniseikonia that he could perform using his Bausch & Lomb Greens' Refractor.[1] The additional equipment included Keystone aniseikonia cards, a septum to separate the views of the two sides of the card to the two eyes, and apparatus to hold the two sides of the test card equidistant from the refractor. The Keystone aniseikonia cards (see Figure A5.1 for an example) were designed to be used with trial lenses in a stereoscope, but that is not how Pratt used them. The following were the steps of his aniseikonia testing:

1) A card from the Keystone aniseikonia set is placed on the reading rod at 16 inches and a septum is suspended from the reading rod so that each side of the card is seen by one eye only.
2) The test is begun with the lenses from the endpoint of the unfused cross cylinder test (OEP 14A) in place.
3) Base-out prism is added in front of both eyes until the two sides appear to be fused into one.
4) The patient should then see one white X, two vertical white lines, and two vertical green lines which appear to be closer than the X. (The green lines are outside of the vertical white lines)
5) The patient is asked whether the left or right green line is closer than the other. Plus sphere is added on the side of the closer green line or minus sphere is added on the side of the farther green line until they appear to be equidistant.

6) The patient is asked if the left or right side of the X appears closer than the other. Over the eye on the same side as the closer side of the X, the examiner can (a) add minus cylinder axis 180, or (b) reduce minus cylinder axis 90, or (c) turn the minus cylinder axis toward 180. Alternatively, the examiner could reduce minus cylinder axis 180 or add minus cylinder axis 90 over the eye on the same side as the farther side of the X. Any of those changes are made until the two sides of the X appear equidistant.
7) The patient is asked if the top or bottom of the X appears closer than the other. If the bottom is closer, the examiner can (a) rotate the right eye minus cylinder axis from 180 toward 135 and the left eye minus cylinder axis from 180 toward 45, or (b) if the minus cylinder axes are greater than 90 and less than 180 in the right eye and 1 or greater and less than 90 in the left eye, minus cylinder power can be increased, or (c) if the minus cylinder axes are 1 or greater and less than 90 in the right eye and greater than 90 and less than 180 in the left eye, minus cylinder power can be decreased. If the top of the X seems closer, the examiner can (a) rotate the right eye minus cylinder axis from 180 toward 45 and the left eye minus cylinder axis from 180 toward 135, or (b) if the minus cylinder axes are less than 180 and more than 90 in the right eye and 1 or greater and less than 90 in the left eye, minus cylinder can be decreased, or (c) if minus cylinder axes are 1 or greater and less than 90 in the right eye and less than 180 and greater than 90 in the left eye, minus cylinder power can be increased.
8) If the two green lines appear equidistant to the patient, the two sides of the X appear equidistant, and the top and bottom of the X appear equidistant, the sphere, cylinder axis for each eye in the refractor are recorded.
9) The test card is turned over so that if the number 18 was on the top as in Figure A5.1, now the 18 is on the bottom.
10) Steps 4 through 8 are repeated.

Pratt's Method of Aniseikonia Measurement

Pratt then used those findings to calculate the amount of aniseikonia expressed as an interocular magnification difference. The following are the calculations that he performed:

1) Break cylinders down into their 90/180 and 45/135 components using the graph in either Figure 4.3 or Figure 4.4.
2) Express the findings as interocular spherical equivalent difference, an interocular difference in cylinder power in either axis 90 or axis 180, and an interocular difference in cylinder power in either axis 45 or axis 135 for each side of the card. (One side of the card gives the interocular magnification difference plus the magnification difference in the card. The other side of the card gives the interocular magnification difference minus the magnification difference in the card.)
3) Add each of the interocular differences for the two sides of the card and divide by two. This will give the interocular magnification difference.
4) Subtract each of the interocular differences for one side of the card from their corresponding differences for the other side of the card and divide by two. This should give the magnification difference in the card and should be close to the difference printed on the back of the card.
5) Break the P-factors for the right and left eyes down into spherical equivalents and the 90/180 and 45/135 components of the cylinder. Find the interocular difference for each of those three numbers.
6) Find the differences between the eikonometric interocular differences and the P-factor interocular differences for spherical equivalent, 90/180 cylinder component, and 45/135 cylinder component.
7) Using Figure A5.2, convert those interocular dioptric differences into interocular magnification differences.

An interocular magnification difference in the spherical equivalent indicates an overall aniseikonia that can potentially be managed by adjustments in the base curve, vertex distance, and lens thickness of the spectacle lenses, using charts available in the literature.[2,3] An interocular magnification difference in the cylinder components indicates a meridional aniseikonia. Pratt noted that approaches for dealing with meridional aniseikonia included putting opposite sign cylinders on the front and back surfaces of the spectacle lenses or making small adjustments in the cylinder axis prescribed (small enough that visual acuity would not be significantly affected).[1]

References

1. Pratt CB. Presentations and demonstrations in Aniseikonia Special Clinic, Pacific University, February-April, 1974.
2. Bartlett JD. Anisometropia and aniseikonia. In: Amos JF, ed. Diagnosis and Management in Vision Care. Boston: Butterworths, 1987:173-202.
3. Rayner AW. Aniseikonia and magnification in ophthalmic lenses: Problems and solutions. Am J Optom Arch Am Acad Optom 1966;43:617-632.

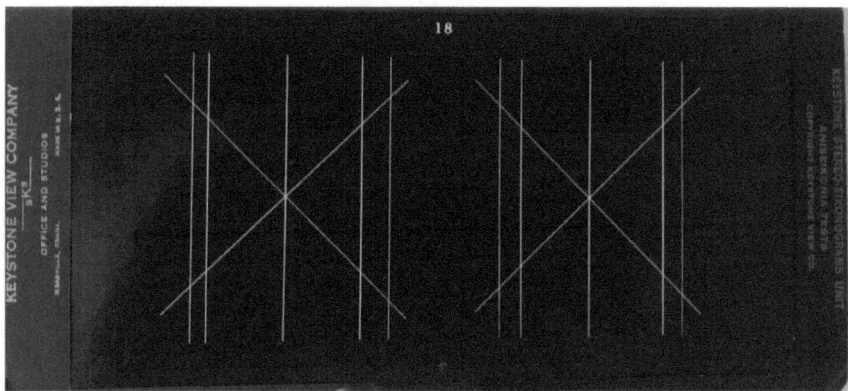

Figure A5.1. An example of the Keystone aniseikonia cards used by Pratt in his aniseikonia testing procedure. Pratt placed the card on the Greens' Refractor reading rod and suspended a septum from the reading rod so that the left side of the card was seen by the left eye and the right side of the card by the right eye. Base-out prism was then added in the Refractor until the views on the two sides of the card were fused by the patient. (From a photograph taken by David Goss)

Figure A5.2. Graph drawn by Pratt to convert the differences between the eikonometric dioptric findings he got from his aniseikonia testing and the anisometropic dioptric findings from the P-factor into interocular magnification differences (diopters on the x-axis and percent magnification on the y-axis). Separate lines show the conversion for different vertex distances in mm. (From a handout distributed by Pratt)

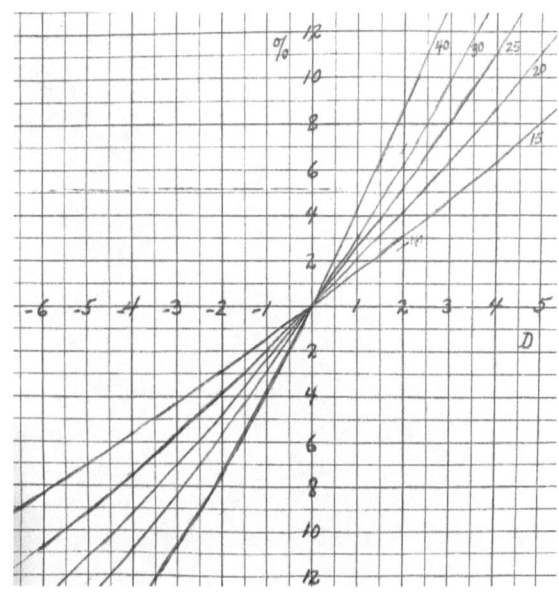

Appendix 6

Carol B. Pratt Scholarship

The Carol B. Pratt Scholarship Fund was established in the 1980s. It was set up by Pratt's sister, Norabel Pratt Miller, and donations have been made, and continue to be made by friends and admirers of Pratt and the university. Scholarships are awarded to entering optometry students for financial assistance during their first year of optometry school. The number and the amounts of the scholarships vary dependent on the earnings of the endowment, with awards of around $2,400 to $2,500 in recent years at the time of this writing. Donations can be made by going to the following link or scanning the QR code below: www.pacificu.edu/give/make-gift-carol-pratt-endowed-scholarship-fund

About the Authors

The authors are alumni of the Pacific University College of Optometry. David Goss has enjoyed a long career in academic optometry at Northeastern State University in Oklahoma and Indiana University. Among his previous books are *Ocular Accommodation, Convergence, and Fixation Disparity*, *Clinical Management of Myopia*, *Introduction to the Optics of the Eye*, and *From Spectacle Making Trade to Scholarly Profession: A History of Optometry in the United States*. He has served as editor of *Hindsight: Journal of Optometry History* since 1995. Scott Pike practiced optometry for over 30 years in Montana and Oregon, and he has been an optometry faculty member for over 20 years at Southern California College of Optometry and Pacific University. He is a past president of the Pacific University Alumni Association, and he received Pacific University's Outstanding Alumni Award in 2020. He has run a non-profit eye care project, Enfoque Ixcán, in rural Guatemala since 1997.

www.ingramcontent.com/pod-product-compliance
Lightning Source LLC
Chambersburg PA
CBHW030337100526
44592CB00010B/722